Vitamin D

Health Benefits and Healing Powers of
Vitamin D

*(Health Benefits and Cure for Depression and
Diabetes)*

George Smith

Published By **John Kembrey**

George Smith

*Vitamin D: Health Benefits and Healing Powers
of Vitamin D (Health Benefits and Cure for
Depression and Diabetes)*

ISBN 978-1-77485-461-7

Legal & Disclaimer

The information contained in this book is not designed to replace or take the place of any form of medicine or professional medical advice. The information in this book has been provided for educational and entertainment purposes only.

The information contained in this book has been compiled from sources deemed reliable, and it is accurate to the best of the Author's knowledge; however, the Author cannot guarantee its accuracy and validity and cannot be held liable for any errors or omissions. Changes are periodically made to this book. You must consult your doctor or get professional medical advice before using any of the suggested remedies, techniques, or information in this book.

TABLE OF CONTENTS

Introduction

Recent studies suggest that up to 77 percent of Americans have a deficiency with the vitamin D. Vitamin D may be one of the less known, yet the most vital nutrients that one need to supplement every day. It is often known as the "sunshine vitamin" this vitamin is fat-soluble vitamin and belongs to the same family as vitamins D-2 as well as D-3. One of the most important roles for vitamin D that it allows the body to effectively to absorb calcium and phosphorus. This is often neglected because many people think that vitamin B is easily available through spending time in the sunlight. Although it is true that the interaction of UV rays with the skin can produce vitamin D, supplementation will ensure that you do not be afflicted by a variety of health-related issues. With people today spending longer and longer in the indoors it's difficult for our bodies to produce all the different components of vitamin D it needs. In addition, poor health can limit the quantity of vitamin D, and the right amount required to ensure healthy health. Vitamin D is essential for the development of strong bones.

This is especially important for those over 50 as well as youngsters during their development age. In addition, vitamin D vital for your health but new studies are being conducted each day to prove its effects on moods as well as the reduction of depression. With millions of people on antidepressants, it's possible that all one requires is to add high-quality vitamin D in order to combat the negative depressive effects. There are other reasons that you should think about eating vitamin D, that we will explore in this fascinating and informative guide. Make sure you go through this book as the knowledge and information gained from studying vitamin D could last all your life and enhance every day!

Chapter 1: Explains What Does It Mean To Be Vitamin D?

Vitamin D is among the essential nutrients your body requires every day. Its effect goes beyond the fact that it makes your teeth and bones stronger. Vital organs require vitamin D to function properly. The body also requires it to fight off infections.

Many people believe that vitamin D is a product of the sun. It's not. The reason sun exposure is beneficial is that it triggers certain substances on the skin which are responsible for creating vitamin D. Yes, the body has the ability to produce the vitamin D it needs. This is what makes this vitamin different among all other vitamins.

Vitamin D is also obtainable by eating food items. It is also taken in supplements. The intake of vitamin D is crucial to ensure that your body is healthy.

Vitamin D is a synthesis product of sun exposure

In particular more specifically, the UVB radiations from the sun are those that trigger vitamin D synthesizing. It is a process that requires wavelengths of 300-320 nanometers. The wavelength is able to be absorbed by the skin (not protected by sunscreen lotions or clothing). Once it penetrates the skin's deeper layer, it converts the 7-dehydrocholesterol compound on the skin into vitamin D. This process will take another set of steps before it becomes the bio-available vitamin D3.

Certain aspects can influence the degree to which UVB gets into the skin and, consequently, the amount of vitamin D3 is produced in the human body. The cloud cover (complete) decreases the energy derived from UVB by 50 percent. Shade can reduce the power that is UVB by 60 percentage. This is not only limited to the blocking of sunlight caused by an airborne pollution (particulates). Glass doesn't allow UVB to enter through. So, sun exposure in indoor areas (i.e. the sunlight that streams through the glass of a window) does not trigger vitamin D synthesizing. Sunscreens with SPF 8 or above blocks UVB.

The duration of exposure to the sun will also influence the amount of vitamin D is synthesized. The most common recommendation is that sun exposure of five to 30 minutes at least twice every week is efficient in stimulating sufficient vitamin D production to satisfy the body's requirements. It is recommended to expose yourself during the hours of 10 AM until 3 PM. Skin on back legs arm, face or arms are the best places to be exposed to the sun without sunscreen.

Supplementation is recommended for those who are not able to get this type of sunlight exposure.

Making vitamin D on your own is the best. If exposed to sunlight that is reflected off the skin, skin-related compounds become active and begin the process of the process of natural Vitamin D synthesis. The resultant compound will be vitamin D3. It is bioavailable and is easily absorbs by all tissues within the body.

Vitamin D3 sulfate is an final outcome of vitamin D production in the human body. The supplements contain also vitamin D3 however, in unsulfated form. When it is sulfated vitamin D3 is water-soluble, which makes it more likely to circulate in blood. The form that is not sulfated needs bad LDL cholesterol to circulate through blood.

It also has other advantages. When face is exposed sunlight it not only triggers vitamin D synthesizing. The sun also stimulates creation of large quantities of cholesterol sulfate. This compound plays an essential part in maintaining the heart's health and all the other parts of our cardiovascular system. According to research conducted by Dr. Stephanie Seneff, low levels of cholesterol sulfate can be related to elevated concentrations of LDL (bad cholesterol) and heart disease. In addition, low levels of cholesterol can trigger growth of various diseases like obesity and diabetes.

Another reason is that there isn't an excess dosage to take when taking Vitamin D through sun exposure. The body has the ability to regulate its processes to ensure that levels remain within the normal levels.

What is the process? Vitamin D is utilized by the body

The principal purpose that this vitamin has is the regulation of the quantity of calcium that is present in our bodies. This is impacting many different processes.

When skin is exposed to sunlight Vitamin D precursors within the skin get activated. This is also the beginning of the process that is involved in vitamin D synthesis. The activated substance within the skin is then transferred directly to liver. Vitamin D from foods and supplements are processed by the digestive tract and then sent to the liver.

Within the liver, vitamin D gets transformed into 25(OH)D. As such, vitamin D is able to be circulated via bloodstream and transported to the kidneys.

The kidneys are the organ of which further steps take place to make active vitamin D. In this way vitamin D can be utilized by the tissues.

Vitamin D that is activated can be used in two ways:

* By controlling calcium levels in the bones, the gut, and blood.

* Helping to facilitate more efficient as well as efficient communications between cells of the body

Special population

There are different requirements at various stages and in different conditions. Breastfeeding and pregnant women generally require more attention due to their bodies engaged in a variety of tasks. Their health is also a factor in the health of the growing foetus as well as the breastfeeding baby as it pertains to. In accordance with the Health Department, vitamin D intake guidelines for these particular instances are:

* All lactating and pregnant women must take vitamin D supplements daily. The recommended daily dosage is 0.01 mg (10 micrograms). This amount will satisfy the requirements of the mother and allow the foetus to develop his own vitamin D reserves the baby will require in early infancy.

* All infants and children ranging aged 6 months up to five years old need to be taking supplements every day with Vitamin D droplets. This can help them attain the optimal vitamin D levels determined for their age group. The intake amount is 0.007 up to 0.0085 mg (7 to 8 micrograms).

For infants fed formula Vitamin D drops are not needed since the majority of infant formulas already come enriched with essential minerals and vitamins. But, if your infant consumes less than 500 milliliters or around a pint of the formula each day, their vitamin intake might not be sufficient. Vitamin D supplementation (in quantities similar to those above and appropriate for their age) is then required.

* Infants breastfeeding may require vitamin D supplementation. The supplementation would begin at 1 month old. This would be applicable even if the mother hasn't taken Vitamin D supplements during her pregnancy.

For adults, a daily vitamin D intake in the amount of 0.01 mg (10 micrograms) is required in any of the following situations:

* Over 65 years old

* Covers the skin in line with traditional practices

* Spends long hours in the indoors, for example, those who live in a house or housebound

The history of Vitamin D

The findings and subsequent research regarding vitamin D are tightly linked to the treatment and study of rickets, an illness caused by a lack of this vitamin within the body.

This crucial chemical behaves as an hormone. The first discovery and the classification of this chemical as a vitamin was an accidental. Sir Edward Mellanby was studying dogs from 1919 until 1920. The dogs were raised in a dark, secluded area and were not exposed to sunlight to any way. The study was aimed at establishing an appropriate diet that would show that rickets is caused by the lack of the trace vitamin. He published his findings in 1921. released his findings.

It was concluded by the researcher that fats play an important role in the development of rickets most likely due to an accessory vitamin or food item which could be similar to the fat-soluble vitamin. Sir Mellanby's research was successful in establishing the fact that cod liver oil functions as an excellent antirachitic medication.

The next study focused the vitamin. E.V. McCollum and his colleagues were able to discern the distinction between Vitamin A as well as Vitamin D. Vitamins that are fat-soluble preparations were exposed to bubbling oxygen. This led to the deactivation of vitamin A, while vitamin D remained active.

A study that was conducted during 1923 Golblatt and Soames discovered the vitamin D precursor in the skin's structure. This compound was called 7-dehydrocholesterol. The researchers also discovered that irradiating the compound with UV radiation or light resulted in the substance that was similar to fat-soluble vitamins. Further research on this was carried out by Weinstock and Hess. Their study proved that UV light can produce vitamin D. In this study, a tiny skin part was extracted and split in two. One part was irradiated and the other wasn't. Then, the irradiated portions were fed to rats with rachitic diseases. The results showed that the skin was able to shield against rickets, whereas non-irradiated skin did not.

Another study carried out by Steenbock and Black further examined the trace element. The study revealed that the element in question was not a food item and was something the body was able to create. At the time when nutrition science was on the rise. This led for the development of water-soluble and fat-soluble vitamins. In turn, an antirachitic protein (which will later be referred to in the future as vitamin D) was swiftly identified as an vitamin.

In the 1930s, nature of the chemical formula in vitamin D was discovered in the 1930s. This was due to an effort of a group headed by Prof. Adolf Otto Reinhold Windaus in Germany at a lab located at the University of Gottingen. Windaus thoroughly studied the vitamin, and it was known"the Vitamin D project. He collaborated with over fifty postdoctoral or doctoral scientists. His team's work led to him receiving a Nobel Prize in Chemistry, because of his work in studying the connection between sterols as well as vitamins.

It was in 1932 that the chemical features that vitamin D2 were discovered. It was a type of vitamin D which is produced by exposing ergosterol to UV radiation. It wasn't until the year 1936 when vitamin D3 could be chemically identified. This form can be made by submitting 7-dehydrcholesterol to UV radiation. This was during the identification of the antirachitic component in cod liver oil that was first examined by the scientist Sir Mellanby. It was this compound which prompted the research on Vitamin D. The study discovered that the antirachitic chemical was similar with vitamin D3. The chemical structure suggested it was a steroid, specifically a seco-steroid.

Health benefits from Vitamin D

The most widely-publicized benefits of Vitamin D are prevention of rickets among children. In the past, and in many studies vitamin D is widely recognized as a crucial factor in healthy living. Its significance is not is limited to bones. The benefits of this supplement extend to other organs as well as various elements of health.

The vast array of advantages is facilitated by the distinct activity that this vitamin. When vitamin D is bioavailable, it's transformed into a hormone-like substance. This is usually referred to as the calcitriol form or activated vitamin D.

The decades of research have shown numerous benefits to growing the amount of vitamin D within the body, particularly that of D3. A large number of chronic illnesses that result in around one million deaths every year could be avoided by simply increasing levels of vitamin D in the body.

Cancer risk reduction

Simply by increasing the amount of vitamin D3 in blood, your risk of breast cancer is decreased. This is the conclusion of the study of nurses conducted by Nurses' Health Study. The reduction in cancer risk was seen in nurses with the most levels of vitamin D3 blood levels, which was the average 50ng/mL. Risk reduction was around 50 percent.

Another study conducted in Canada produced similar results. Women who received the greatest exposure to sunlight in their teens and early adulthood had nearly 70% lower risk of breast cancer.

Some additional studies have confirmed the benefits. Increased levels that vitamin D is present in blood decreases the risk of developing colorectal cancer, prostate cancer, and other fatal kinds of cancer. Vitamin D assists in keeping the integrity of cells as well as regulating the growth of cells. This is a huge help in keeping the growth of cancer at the minimal.

Vitamin D can also help boost the immune system. It regulates the expression of various genes that regulate the process of forming an immune system. They specifically affect immune cells by telling that they must fight and kill invaders like bacteria and viruses.

Help protect the your cardiovascular system

Vitamin D provides protection and beneficial functions for the heart and other parts part of the cardiovascular system. It can lower blood pressure, prevent the development of atherosclerotic heart disease stroke, heart attack and stroke. People who lack the vitamin increase their chances of suffering from heart disease by up to 50 percent. The people who have low levels of vitamin D have the highest chance of dying from a heart attack.

Autoimmune disorders

Vitamin C is an efficient modulator of all the functions of immune cells. These functions make it an extremely important component for the prevention and treatment of autoimmune diseases. The research has shown positive results in the treatment of autoimmune diseases like IBD (inflammatory intestinal disease) and MS with Vitamin D supplementation.

Combat Infection

Due to its powerful impact over the immune system's function, Vitamin D is able to boost the body's capacity to fight off infections. This includes all types of diseases, such as influenza. Vitamin D can also be involved to the production of over 200 peptides which possess vital antimicrobial effects within the body. This is among the major reasons why vitamin D is so efficient against common illnesses like colds and flu.

A study in Japan which involved schoolchildren demonstrated the effectiveness of vitamin D in preventing infections. In the study, students received vitamin D at 1,200 units a day throughout winter. The children had a lower risk of developing influenza A by as high as 40 percent. This makes it a less risky and more effective method to protect vulnerable populations from flu rather than getting a vaccine. Flu vaccines can cause certain issues, particularly for those with egg allergies.

Increased metabolism and repair of DNA

A study conducted by Dr. Holick found that vitamin D enhances metabolic processes through enhancing the body's capacity in repairing DNA. The study found that the daily intake of vitamin D for a period of time resulted in the increase in regulation of 291 genes. These genes were responsible for the metabolic processes of up to 80 within the body. One of these processes is responsible for decreasing autoxidation. It is an process of oxidation that occurs when there is UV radiation or oxygen. Autoxidation plays an important role in the formation of cancer as well as in the process of aging.

Protection against chronic illnesses

No matter what gender, health condition or age, consuming the proper amount and amount of vitamin D can reduce the chance of developing a diverse range of chronic illnesses such as common ailments, sex and age. health issues like:

* Hypertension

* Obesity

* Type 1 Diabetes (Type 1 as well as Type)

* Autism

* Crohn's disease

* Rheumatoid arthritis

* Insomnia

* Tuberculosis

* Multiple Sclerosis

* Cavities

* Septicemia

* Dementia

* Muscle pain

* Inflammatory colon disease

* Hearing loss

* Age-related signs

* Psoriasis

* Periodontal disease

* Eczema

* Infertility

* Reduced risk of C-section (for pregnant women who are taking Vitamin D supplementation)

* Osteoporosis

* Asthma

* Seizures

* Macular degeneration

* Migraines

* Pre-eclampsia

* Cystic Fibrosis

* Depression

* Schizophrenia

* Alzheimer's disease

Vitamin D Deficiency

People who do not receive enough vitamin D daily may suffer from vitamin D deficiencies. Many suffer from this problem. Even infants are susceptible to vitamin D deficiencies.

For many years in the past, the medical and scientific community believed that 20 nanograms of vitamin D in a milliliter blood to be sufficient to satisfy the needs of the tissues. The latest research indicates that the body requires at 30 ng/mL to be healthy and in good health.

If the issue isn't taken care of immediately, it could cause your life to be at risk.

The only reliable way to know if someone is suffering from vitamin D deficiency is to conduct tests on blood. There are however a few indicators and signs that could inform a person of the presence of the deficiencies. If you notice any of these symptoms you should be sure to consult a physician and have the appropriate testing to confirm the diagnosis and prompt treatment.

RISKS FOR VITAMIN D DEFICIENCY

Certain conditions put a person at a greater chance of having vitamin D deficiencies.

Dark skin

Skin that is darker at a higher risk of developing Vitamin D deficiency. The dark skin color is a result of melanin pigments that are more abundant on the skin's layers. This forms a protective layer which blocks sunlight and shields the more fatty layer of skin. This is a defense mechanism but it could have a negative effect on vitamin D production. Because of the more dense melanin layer of dark skin, there is less sunlight to reach the skin and trigger the process of vitamin D synthesizing. This results in a decrease in the capacity to make sufficient vitamin D. For those with dark skin, they require 10 times longer exposed to sunlight to make the appropriate quantities of vitamin D.

Vitamin D production by the skin that is activated through sun exposure is the primary source of this vital vitamin. If your body is having difficulties producing it, there's more chance of being deficient.

Too little sun exposure

Insufficient sun exposure is also a significant chance of the development of deficiency syndromes. Many people avoid the sun due to the adverse effects of sun exposure. It causes premature ageing, dark spots, sunburns, wrinkles and wrinkles. There is also the risk of skin cancer from excessive sun exposure. In addition to these concerns is the danger of getting too much.

Be sure to check your location to determine the best times for exposure to the sun. In general, exposure to the sun between 6AM and 10AM is fine and doesn't cause much harm in comparison to exposure to midday sun.

Living in northern latitudes

According to several studies people who live in northern latitudes are at a higher risk of having vitamin D deficiencies. Northern latitude is regions located north of the 37th parallel. According to research that have been conducted, the angle of sun's rays in winter months isn't enough to create the force required to trigger vitamin D synthesizing. To confirm this, research shows that the majority of people within these areas have low levels of vitamin D within their bloodstreams, with the most low levels occur during winter months.

Vegan diet

The vegan diet could be an ideal choice due to the numerous advantages of eating vegetables and fruits. But, this type of diet can lead to deficiency in vitamin D. The diet is a way to eliminate the foods that are high in vitamin D. These usually come from animals. Some examples include liver oil and the fatty fishes. These foods are excellent sources of vitamin D. Vegan diets do not permit these food items. This could pose a possibility for deficiency conditions.

Achy bones

Many people are mistakenly diagnosed by a condition called chronic fatigue syndrome, or fibromyalgia, when they visit a physician for the pain and aches. Many of the symptoms that are associated with these conditions are a classic sign for Vitamin D deficiency. Insufficient amounts of vitamin D within the body can cause inadequate absorption of calcium in the collagen matrix of bone. This causes the painful throbbing sensation that is felt across the bones. If left untreated the bone structure is likely to shrink, triggering the development of diseases such as osteoporosis.

Head sweating

It is one of the first signs that show up, particularly among newborns. If a baby's head begins to sweat excessively or abnormally sweaty, mothers should examine their infant for deficiency in vitamin D. The excessive sweating may be caused by neuromuscular irritation due to the lack of vitamin D.

The weakness of muscles and joints and muscle pain

It is also important to note that the importance of vitamin B for the musculoskeletal system cannot to be undervalued. Inadequate levels of this vitamin could hinder the performance and endurance of muscles and joints. Deficiency may cause weakness and pain to these organs.

Tiredness or fatigue

Because bones and muscles aren't well-nourished and nourished, they are easily fatigued. Vitamin D assists minerals get into these organs, so they function at optimal levels. If vitamin D is not present, the performance and endurance decreases significantly which can cause fatigue.

Vitamin D Overdose

On the other hand, individuals are also susceptible to suffering from an overdose of vitamin D. It is also known as vitamin D toxicity or hypervitaminosis. Any excess of anything is harmful for health regardless of whether it's an excess of the essential nutrients. There isn't a rule of thumb that says "the more the better" in the realm of health.

The positive side is the fact that vitamin D overdose is not common because our bodies have their own internal regulatory checkpoint that prevents an excessive accumulation and toxication of nutrients within the body.

What can you tell if are taking too many Vitamin D

The blood test is the most reliable method to determine if the intake is excessive. It is the 25(OH)D levels in blood will be checked. Tests that show more than 150 ng/mL have been identified as potentially harmful, and can cause the potential for harm to health. Toxicity is confirmed when a high 25(OH)D result is associated with significant levels of calcium present in blood.

Who is at risk of the overdose of vitamin D?

In the event of taking large doses, it do not instantly place a person at risk of risk of overdose since the body is naturally able to eliminate excess amounts or store it in the fat tissues. But, it is dependent on the body's overall capacity and general health.

Children are at a higher risk of being overdosed in vitamin D supplementation. To decrease the risk, you must follow these guidelines:

* Children who weigh less than 25 pounds should not consume vitamin D supplements more than 500.000 IU in a single day, or more than 2 000 IU daily for more than 3 months.

* Children who weigh between 25 and 50 pounds should not consume vitamin D supplements that exceed 100,000 units in 24 hours or more than 4,000IU per day for longer than 3 months.

* Children who weigh between 50 and 75 pounds shouldn't take vitamin D supplements that exceed 150,000 IU within 24 hours , or over 6, 000 IU each day for longer than 3 months.

* Children who weigh between 75 and 100 pounds shouldn't take vitamin D supplements that exceed 200 000 IU in less than 24 hours, or more than 8 1,000 IU daily for more than three months.

What happens if you take an the case of overdose?

Overdose is not a thing that happens immediately. It is not within a couple of hours following the intake of the once-in-a-lifetime dosage of vitamin D. It will develop gradually, as a result of daily large doses of supplements. The body naturally stores excess unabsorbed or inactive vitamin D in the fat tissues. If the fats' storage capacity is exhausted, that is the time when symptoms begin to manifest. When symptoms start to show the levels are already thought to be toxic, and treatment must be initiated immediately.

When amounts of vitamin D get excessively overly high in the body, it will begin to produce the chemical 25(OH)D. When the levels of vitamin D continue increase, 25(OH)D levels also increase in blood. This is how test for Vitamin D overdose and toxicity detect.

What are the signs of an overdose?

The primary result of an vitamin D overdose is an excess concentration of calcium in the blood. This is known as hypercalcemia. This can put your body at risk of more serious issues.

If there is hypercalcemia, the following signs and symptoms can be seen:

* feeling or being sick

* Feeling very thirsty

* Loss of appetite

* poor appetite

* frequent urination

* abdominal discomfort

* constipation or diarrhea

* Bone pain

* muscle weakness or pain

* Feeling tired

* Feeling confused

In the blood, excessive levels of calcium could lead to a serious situation. The kidneys are awash with calcium and can cause severe damage to.

In addition, having too much vitamin D in blood could have a negative impact on bones and calcium deposits. In normal quantities vitamin D can encourage the entry of calcium into bones. However, the opposite happens when there is excessive vitamin D in the blood. It will pull calcium deposits from the matrix of bone. This weakens the bones and make them more brittle.

Vitamin D Supplements vs Diet

In order to get the proper quantity of Vitamin D extremely vital. It is also important to note that it is important to note that the RDA for this essential vitamin amounts to 600 mg daily. As mentioned previously there are three primary methods to obtain vitamin D. This is through sunlight exposure (which stimulates vitamin D synthesis which happens naturally within the body) supplementation, and food.

Supplements and diets can increase your levels of vitamin D within the body. The issue is which is more effective - food or supplements? Which is more beneficial in meeting the body with vitamin D?

Vitamin D supplements

Oral supplements typically contain the same type of vitamin D that is the one that is naturally synthesized by the body after exposure to sunlight. Make sure you purchase one that provides the recommended dose of vitamin D in the form of D3 and not in the D2 form.

The benefit of supplementing with vitamin D is that they offer higher quantities than food. It is possible to get as high as 2000 IU or more in one pill. It's also simpler to take. It's just one pill and all of your vitamin D requirements are already taken care of.

Another benefit of supplements is that vitamin D is easily absorbed by your body. It's already in the state where it'll need a few steps to make the vitamin bioavailable.

Vitamin D-rich foods

Certain foods can be great source of vitamins D in nature. But even the highest vitamin D-rich food items have tiny amounts in comparison to the body's demands. For example, if you decide to get the bulk of your body's vitamin D requirements from eggs, you'll need to consume around 10 eggs (or more) during all day.

Yet, adding vitamins D-rich food items is beneficial to include in everyday meals. However, relying solely on food to help you get enough vitamin D isn't a good option.

If you decide to choose the right food sources to meet the daily Vitamin D requirements You have the option of the source of vitamin D: plants or from animal sources. Animal-based sources can provide D3. Plant-based sources can supply people with vitamin D2. Therefore, it's preferential to obtain D2 from sources that are animal-based. Examples include:

Vitamin D2 as well as D3

Supplements may have Vitamin D2 as well as vitamin D3. Vitamin D2 is a synthetic ingredient in supplements. produced and is referred to as ergocalciferol. This type of supplement is produced by exposing plant matter and fungal matter to radiation. This kind of supplement is the one prescribed by the majority of medical professionals. But, it's nowhere as effective as the one that is produced by the body when it is exposed to light.

Vitamin D3 supplements are known as cholecalciferol. It is exactly like the vitamin naturally produced by the body. A meta-analysis has found that there is a distinction in the results obtained from these two different kinds of supplements. Users who took D3 supplements saw an increase of 6% in risk. The people who used D2 had an increase of 2% in risk of adverse reactions.

For many years, D2 and D3were considered to be quite alike and could be utilized interchangeably. This was based on older research that looked at rickets in infants, and the importance of vitamin D in the treatment.

In the present, research has yielded more recent results which lead to a greater comprehension of the role of vitamin D. These findings showed that there was a substantial distinction in the 2.

Research has shown studies have shown that D3 is 87 percent more efficient than D2. It increases and maintains levels of vitamin D in the blood more efficiently. It also is better at producing a 2 to 3 times increase in the storage of vitamin D.

Another study has found that the shelf-life for vitamin D2 is very short. It breaks down quickly and, most likely, when someone takes it, the supplement will already have lost the majority of its potency.

In the body the metabolites that make up Vitamin D are also not as effective in bringing the benefits that we want. They have a weak binding actions with proteins within the body. The compounds are not circulated or taken in by the body.

Whatever shape the supplement is in, it must be transformed by the body to make use of the tissues. D3 supplements are converted at a the speed of D2 supplements, up to 500% more quickly.

Reference Intakes

The Food and Nutrition Board or FNB has set up the RDA (Recommended Daily Allowance) for vitamin D. The RDA is the amount of daily intake of vitamin D per day to fulfill the nutritional needs for the 97-98% healthy adults.

* Infants between 0 and 12 months old (both both female and male) 400IU (or 10 mg

* Children aged 1-18 year old (both both female and male) 500 IU, or 15 mg

* Females 14-18 year old who is pregnant or lactating (600 IU) or 15 mg

* 19 - the age of 50 (both genders) 600 IU, or 15 mcg

* Females aged 19- 50 years old, who are pregnant or lactating: 600 IU or 15 mg

* Between 51 and 70 year old (both both) 600 IU, or 15 mg

* More than age 70 (both both) 800 IU, or 20 mg

Chapter 2: How Vitamin D Deficiency Is Like

If you are unable to go out into the outside due to problems with allergies, that supplementing with vitamin D is a great idea. Vitamin D deficiency could result and put a lot of us at risk , even in the absence of any indication. Aversion to sun exposure is only one aspect which could cause deficiency. There are other aspects that ought to be thinking about in addition such as: * Allergies to milk - many folks are well aware of the fact that not all product is enriched with vitamin D, so this could be a good source. The presence of milk allergies could lead to the removal of this method of including vitamin D into your diet. * Vegan diets - though there are numerous health advantages to eating a vegan diet generally, vegans do not consume any products. Avoidance of hormones - the majority of people know that milk contains added hormones from cows that were injecting and then release these hormones into their milk. A simple way to locate sources of milk like co-ops, Amish milk farms etc. Naturally occurring food items like liver oils, fish and egg yolks may include vitamin D-rich foods to your diet to ensure that you won't be deficient. Kidneys and intestines have problems converting vitamin D some medical conditions, such as Crohn's disease may decrease levels of vitamin D taken in by the body. As you get older, your kidneys might have difficulty processing vitamin D, so supplements may be required. Dark skin - based on the colour of your skin, it will determine the amount of vitamin D the body produces in the sun. * Obesity or BMI higher than 30 percent - those who are overweight usually have less vitamin D levels. It's a great option to supplement your vitamin D levels for those who fall into this category since it could help you shed weight. Signs are a sign of deficiency in vitamin D.

The following lists are signs of vitamin D deficiencies and as you can see , many or a lot of them are typical in the majority of people: * Being sick or experiencing infections frequently If you get frequently sick, especially with flu or colds most likely you've got an insufficient amount of vitamin D. The vitamin D's main functions is to strengthen the immune system. Tiredness and fatigue that is excessive This is a typical problem that is frequently not recognized as a typical issue that many suffer from. However, in the majority of studies, especially among women fatigue and tiredness was due to extremely low levels of vitamin D. * Depression - There have been numerous studies that have shown an improvement or noticeable improvement in moods of people and lessening of depression after they started to take vitamin D supplements. It was also the case when it came to seasonal affective disorder or prolonged periods in colder seasons. * Bone pain could be the most obvious indicator for vitamin D deficiency, where your bones are aching. It is more common among the elderly and must be monitored closely. The lower back is a common cause of pain. lower back pain extremely common in vitamin D deficiencies. Studies have revealed that older women may experience increased levels of pain in the back during physical activities. • Slower or less effective healing. wound healing - similar to diabetics experiencing problems closing wounds. A low level of vitamin D could delay or even stop healing and closure of wounds. The loss of bone - commonly known as osteoporosis the decrease in strength or bone disease may eventually cause and create a variety of issues. For instance, people suffering from bone problems can break bones by slipping and fall, whereas an otherwise healthy person who might only suffer a minor bruise. Hair loss is the case that Vitamin D deficiency may cause loss of hair. Alopecia areata can be a type of autoimmune disorder that may cause significant loss of hair across the entire body, and can be linked to the beginning stages of Rickets. * Muscle pain. This is due to muscles cells and their receptors not being stimulated properly by adequate amounts of vitamin D. It is present in children as well as in the elderly. Deficiency can cause excessive sensitivity to pain throughout the body. As you can tell, the availability of vitamin D can be necessary to feel healthy, enjoy less pain, and function effectively day-to-day. Additionally, research has proven that vitamin D plays a significant part in the treatment and/or prevention of many illnesses that are common in our modern society, such as diabetes, insulin resistance, hypertension, and even multiple sclerosis for instance. handful. Testing your level of vitamin D in your blood is the sole method of knowing the current level of your blood. The tests for vitamin D 25-hydroxy. In the next section, remember that you need to be able to achieve 20 nanograms to 50 ng/mL in order to qualify as healthy. If your levels are below 12 n/mL then you're deficient in vitamin D. There are a variety of diseases that could be cured or controlled Through Vitamin D

Since vitamin D acts as a hormone inside the body, it can significantly impact your health and can even stop, control or prevent possible illnesses. It is important to remember that their receptors change your body's requirement for vitamin D. So what makes vitamin D distinct from other vitamins. Let's look at the majority of the most prevalent illnesses and the ways vitamin D may aid in treating cancer The evidence of the numerous benefits of having adequate quantities of vitamin D that help in the treatment of various cancers in the 1980s. Vitamin D has the potential to dramatically affect and confer protection against cancers of the ovarian tract, breast cancer and cancer of the colon. The research is also showing that vitamin D can aid in the prevention or reduction of prostate cancer as well as non-Hodgkin's lymphoma. Vitamin D has been proven in a study conducted in 1993 to improve calcium absorption, to kill cancer cells , and to reduce the growth of cancer. Studies have also pointed to treatments, prevention, and even possible cures. Research continues to reveal the benefits of increasing doses, especially for patients who suffer from cancer of nearly all types. More powerful doses may could lead to curative treatments! Diabetes is a major problem. Millions of people suffer from types I and II of diabetes. The majority of the time, type I is an autoimmune disorder that manifests predominantly in adolescents and children. It affects the body's capacity to make insulin. Vitamin D deficiencies have been proven to be associated with a significant variety of autoimmune diseases and an the increased likelihood of developing the type I diabetes or Type II. Cod liver oil, a method for vitamin D supplements,, especially during the early years of formative years, can help prevent a variety of beneficial effects of inflammation on the body, which could result in diabetes. Osteoporosisis among the most well-known diseases caused by vitamin D deficiency and it is estimated that there are around 25 million people in the United States alone that are susceptible to developing osteoporosis. The cause of the disease is insufficient calcium levels and vitamin D deficiency certainly contributes to the body's inability of absorbing it effectively. Vitamin D is essential in maintaining and sustaining of healthy and strong bones, which is essential to prevent loss of bone especially in those who are elderly. Menopausal women are most at risk and should be taking supplements immediately. As we age, our body's ability to produce vitamin D from Sun exposure. Therefore, supplementation is a must. More than half of all women admitted to hospitals with fractures of the hip or bone-related issues are directly connected to the low amounts in vitamin D. Inflammatory bowel disorders A large percentage of patients suffer from this type of disorder which cause intestinal inflammation. The United States, over 600,000 new cases each year are reported in one way or another. A well-known types is called durable bowel disease or Crohn's disease, which results from the formation of ulcers that develop in both the large and small intestines. There are other conditions that are categorized under this type of illness, but they all have the same thing: the absence of vitamin D. A proper treatment regimen with vitamin D allows the anti-inflammatory process in the body to begin and hormonal changes that slow down and eventually stop the progression of the inflammation-related attacks. Multiple sclerosis: New research has found the direct correlation to the amount of sunlight and whether or not a person is susceptible to developing this disease and how to treat it. Vitamin D is a key part in maintaining and remission of the condition. As you can observe vitamin D isn't simply another vitamin. The tensive cod liver forms or liquid extracts could provide a solution for the control, suppression, and even treatment of these diseases.

Chapter 3: Redefining Your Lifestyle Using Vitamin D

It is now obvious for you to know that advantages of vitamin D extend far beyond the mere fact that you have strong bones. Every study is linking vitamin D to incredible capabilities in the prevention of and possibly curative treatments for autoimmune diseases, cancer and cardiovascular diseases blood pressure issues, alteration of cholesterol levels neurologic disorders, obesity the kidney, reproductive issues, muscle pain, muscles disorders and even a decrease of tooth decay! Vitamin D is definitely a an integral part of your new life style and you should consider taking your time to think about the potential benefits of diseases prevention, disease suppression and the possibility that if you suffer from any of these conditions or illnesses, you might possibly have it treated! How to Change Your Lifestyle with Vitamin D A lot of people want to learn the most effective methods to alter their life to be able to boost the vitamin D levels and overall health. First steps you need to do is figure out precisely what you're doing to ensure your physical health. Healthy people adhere to a certain way of life which includes: * A proper diet, which is full of vitamin D-rich foods. * Regular exercise sufficient to keep and improve your health. Avoiding a lifestyle of sedentary.

Don't use sunscreens (many are harmful anyway). Although most people are aware of these issues however, it's sometimes helpful to understand it in detail. For a healthy lifestyle, it is essential to eat a diet filled with vegetables, quality proteins , and food items that are high in vitamin D, as well as other Micro and macro nutrients. The majority of people today do not get enough nutrients due to the fact that foods produced by large agricultural companies (often known as Big Agra) are highly lacking in vital nutrients. It is essential to buy your food items from cooperatives or local farmers, farmer markets in your area and organic farmers. It is equally important to exercise regularly and consume clean, filtered water that is free of any toxins or contaminants. Pesticides, contaminants and toxins in food items and in water could cause health issues that could lead to vitamin D deficiencies. The synergistic effects of regular exercise , especially when performed outdoors in the sun will improve overall health and well-being and the absorption of vitamin D. It is also important to stay away from a lifestyle of sedentary. Also even if you have to sit for an extended period of the day, you should break up your work and get outside and roll up your sleeves. put on your pants and make sure you soak at least 30 minutes. of sunlight to your body. It is also a part of vitamin D supplementation , which we'll discuss in the future. If you are suffering from health problems such as being obese or diabetic, taking supplements is not just a great idea , but it is essential. Make sure you exercise regularly and seek out opportunities to improve your flexibility and eating a diet that is rich in dark greens, as well as egg and fish proteins. Deficiencies in your health contribute to vitamin D deficiencies. If, for instance, you are overweight, you're not getting enough vitamin D that can help in the regulation of fat. When designing a program, be aware of your current state of well-being and health, and concentrate on obtaining more vitamin D to compensate for. Then, you must think about the importance of relaxing stress in the form of meditation. Meditation can provide many health benefits like reducing the stress level and pressure levels. The reduction of inflammation is essential to Health. When you lower the stress level and cortisol levels, the body also decrease which helps reduce inflammation, and provides other health advantages. Inflammation is by far the essential factor to control your body's inflammation since it can lead to diseases. Research has proven that inflammation is a contributing factor to a variety of ailments including IBS. The decrease in an environment that is prone to inflammation lowers the risk that you'll contract the condition. If you're not getting enough vitamin D in your body, it increases the levels of cortisol and creates "smoldering problems" that could eventually result in a full-blown autoimmune disease. Researchers are connecting stress relief and physical activity that relieves stress like yoga, to better health and well-being. It is possible that yoga could be one of the most beneficial general regimens you can follow for your body, when it comes to reducing stress, as well as mental and physical well-being. It's not unusual for those who practice yoga to live in their 80s attain optimal health. Yoga can be performed at any level of physical fitness and at any age. When you're looking at your exercise routine, think about yoga and relaxation activities like tai chi that have a similar structure to yoga, but more simple to perform. Anything that can reduce the stress levels in your body will help you improve your health over time, particularly if you take supplements by taking vitamin D.

Chapter 4: Vitamin D And Your Primary Health

Being able to maintain the appropriate quantities of vitamin D could drastically alter your life to the positive. It is important to keep in mind that you must mix other nutrients along with vitamin D, as they work in synergy to boost overall health. This is particularly important in the case of many common illnesses or conditions that affect modern society, including Crohn's disease, diabetes or autoimmune disorders, for instance. In the beginning, it is important to be aware that you're deficient in vitamin D and exactly how much at risk of being deficient in the first place. The fact that at the very least three of four people are lacking in vitamin D ought to motivate individuals to seek their levels of vitamin D tested. Do you need to get a blood test? to find out the levels of Vitamin D. It is a good idea to have your levels tested. There are many kinds of tests are available at your usual health grocery shop or pharmacies. Of course, the most reliable method is to test your blood, which is also administered at home and sent to a lab . Results will be available within several days.

The more expensive versions of testing equipment for vitamin D are similar to how diabetics test their blood with the finger puncture method. The devices are available in varying cost and some are very expensive. I recommend that you make use of regular laboratory tests that can be performed at home, then sent to the post office and results sent electronically to you. It is also possible to get the standard blood test in any medical office that may include additional tests. Reading results Should not be: Optimal 25-hydroxyvitamin-D levels are at least 45-50 *ng/ml

Normal levels of 25-hydroxyvitamin D are: 20-50 *ng/ml

Low or deficient levels

* Below 32 *ng/ml

Serious deficiency - seek medical attention! Below 20ng/mL

*Nanograms per Milliliter (ng/mL)Medical tests usually result as the nanograms (ng) for each milliliter (mL). Nanograms are one-billionth of the weight of a Gram. There could be other amounts suggested by health experts. Be aware that the actual amount you receive could depend on your present situation , and the numbers above are generalizations of the current amounts that are accepted. Once you've established the degree of the vitamin D deficiencies, it's much simpler to choose the correct type of supplementation. There are many vitamin D supplements available. or supplements are created equal. The better the quality of the vitamin D, the greater amount of active ingredients ought to be present. Because vitamin companies exist to earn money, they usually add fillers and other inert ingredients, with a small amount in active components. This is the reason why more is not always the best, but the concentration of the ingredient is crucial. Also, you must have an appropriate balance between not enough and excessive vitamin D. The majority of people boost levels of Vitamin D that they drink in winter or when they plan to stay indoors for extended durations of time. The second step is to avoid taking more than 1,000 IU daily as this can cause toxic levels of vitamin D. This could cause weakness and nausea until your body eliminates the excess vitamin D. Before buying any kind or form of vitamin D be sure that the business that sells it has a third-party certification as well as an ability to adhere to high quality standards. Also, you should examine your vitamin D bottles and verify the USP verification seal . This means that the product has passed through an impartial and non-committal quality assessment. You should ensure that the information in the label is the product you are taking. Look around for the highest quality, and this might not always mean the presence of a capsule. Some formulations are also liquid-based, and are contained in suspensions similar to natural Palm oil. The benefits of taking liquids are that they are a good choice because they're metabolized more efficiently in your body and you'll absorb more of vitamin D. The best moment to drink capsules or liquids is after you've eaten food to ensure that vitamin D is digested efficiently in your stomach. There are basically two types of vitamin D that we've discussed in detail the D2 and. Vitamin D is the culmination of both. It is recommended that if you must focus on a particular type of vitamin D which is D3, it should be D3 as it is the most natural form and uses more buyer skin and is easier for your organism to absorb. If you're on an unusual diet that is vegan, for instance a vegetarian diet, you'll likely prefer D2 since it is made mostly from the store-grown mushrooms. Of course , it's best to choose a blend combination of both D2 and. The most effective mixtures are 50-50 and under 1000 IU's but greater than 500 IU's. Regular blood tests will help determine the amount you need to take in order to stay within the ideal range of 45-50 *ng/ml. By balancing the right amount of vitamin D, you can boost your life, particularly by consuming food items that are high in vitamin D as well as an additional dose of sun. This is particularly beneficial when you've had period of relatively low vitamin D levels in your body. Modifying the quantity of vitamin D you consume, it can alter your moods and enable you to take in more vitamin D in situations where the sun isn't as intense and also to decrease vitamin D levels when you spend longer in the sun. It is recommended to take vitamin D supplements to minimum 250 IU so that your body is able to absorb the nutrients it requires. Be aware that too much vitamin D may be stored through fat tissues. By varying dosages over the time you are supplementing, you'll be in control of the way your body's response to supplementation.

* Summertime - the reduction of dosage depends upon the quantity of sunlight exposure and the diet you eat, but generally you can decrease the amount of supplementation when there are longer durations of sun. In the fall, during autumn, you can boost the intake of vitamin D however, you should keep it to a minimum of 1000 IU's. * Winter is that there is the least amount of sunlight , so you can increase your dose dependent on your health and diet and also to control seasonal affective conditions. Now you understand that the most effective overall supplementation is to combine D2 as well as D3. The most effective supplements are aware of this and are just an issue of gradually and gradually introduction of these vitamins into your diet. Be aware that when you start any regimen of supplementation, you must start with the lowest dose and increase it gradually until your

body is able to adjust. This also gives you time to assess how you feel , and this is an excellent source of feedback to determine is the most effective dosage for you. Be aware that high quantities of vitamin D can accumulate in the body, but may also trigger the feeling of fatigue and nausea, as adverse effects. Other side effects of high doses could also cause kidney failure, high levels of calcium in your blood and stomach, constipation, stomach pain and diarrhea. Vitamin D is also able to interact with other medications, such as steroids, or other medicines that are made for the purpose of regulating vitamins D within your metabolic process. If you regularly take steroids it is essential to consult your doctor prior to starting vitamin D as part of your daily routine.

Chapter 5: Vitamin D And Healthful Diet

If you've got the knowledge to measure the amount of vitamin D within your body the next step is the essential components of healthy diets and the best way to boost vitamin D in a safe manner so that you get the proper amount. Supplementation and the role it Plays

It is important to first consider supplements, and the most effective methods to get more of vitamin D into your diet. Make sure you establish the level of vitamin D within your body, so that you are aware of whether you should supplement at all. Here are some areas that you can affect the levels of vitamin D within your body: Sunshine - clearly the most crucial action you can take is to make sure that your skin is exposed to an appropriate amount of exposure to sunlight. It's actually possible to produce the normal amount of vitamin D within your body by merely receiving enough sunlight exposure. Vitamin D is known as the vitamin that shines because it doesn't require a lot of exposure to allow the body to create at minimum 10,000 IU. Fair skinned individuals with a period of around 20 minutes. of exposure will absorb all the core vitamin D they require. Since our bodies produce amount needed, it understands the process to take in and the appropriate quantities, with the remainder being fat-soluble. The quantity of fat-soluble substances is different from person to person which is produced and, as always, we recommend regular tests for blood to determine the you select and the effectiveness of it. Be aware that absorption levels can differ due to the best duration in which you absorb UV radiation should be limited in order to avoid the skin from being damaged. The darker skinned have a greater resistance to sunburn and damaging UV rays, but everyone needs an amount of exposure to make vitamin D-related elements that are vital to our well-being. It is suggested that when you do get sun exposure, it occurs at the best timing of the day in which the sun will be the most hot. You should, however, be sure to limit your exposure to not at least 20-30 minutes, based on the skin's pigmentation. Quality cod liver oil after you've taken test results and determined that a supplementation of your diet is safe One of the most effective alternatives is a top-quality cod liver oil product. 1 teaspoon or 44 International units (IU's) is the recommended dosage . It is recommended to purchase cod liver oil extract which is administered by pouring it into one teaspoon. The other option is gelcaps which have measured in the range of 400 to 600 IU's . These include Omega 3 6, 7, and 9 fats. A few people prefer fermented cod liver oil because it enhances the quality of the product and the health benefits as well as the absorption and digestibility. Sardines are also available, as well as salmon, mackerel, and tuna - in case you're not aware and especially fish kept in captivity are one of the healthiest foods you can consume. The various varieties of fish are very high in vitamin D. You also get the added benefit of having Omega's in your diet, which can assist in preventing various ailments. It is strongly suggested to increase the quantity of fish you consume. Raw milk, which is unpasteurized and is offered by cooperatives has received an unpopular reputation because of its amazing health benefits. In the present, there hasn't been a fatality reported from someone who consumes raw milk, provided that it's at a temperature that is refrigerated. A lot of cooperatives and whole food distribution networks let you buy raw milk. Incorporating this into your diet will not only boost your intake of vitamin D, but it can aid in maintaining an ideal weight, especially when you're older. Many health advantages have been documented from drinking raw milk, but it could be a weight gainer, so be cautious. Egg yolks - eggs are a an extremely well-known source of vitamin D . They are far healthier to consume than what we've been told. If You Should Not Supplement

The regular blood test will reveal the levels of Vitamin D. However, there are instances that you shouldn't take supplements as it's possible to take too much vitamin D and suffer very serious adverse negative effects. If you suffer from tuberculosis, lymphoma, or sarcoidosis D supplements are not advised. However, this doesn't mean you should not spend some time outdoors in the sunshine. Make sure you are aiming for regular levels and ensure that your vitamin D levels and/or bloodwork monitored by a healthcare specialist. Some of the negative consequences of excessive vitamin D are nausea constipation, vomiting, weakening, weight loss, fatigue and headache. Cleaning the body with vitamin D

Vitamin D is a slow process of increasing its doses until it reaches maximum levels, has the ability to cleanse and detoxify for the human body. It is vital to monitor your the levels of vitamin D when you're using vitamin D to aid in the purpose of cleansing and anti-inflammatory procedures. As the quantity of vitamin D grows within your body, you'll experience a detoxification process that occurs during the very first week. Your body's system will eliminate contaminants through your skin and also whenever you go to the bathroom. It is important to ensure that you're not taking too much vitamin D, which is why regular testing is crucial. Be aware that over the course of several weeks, your body will be cleansing itself, and you'll begin to notice certain adverse effectslike a mild disorientation and headaches. Some nausea and sometimes periods of diarrhea. The effects of the side effects will swiftly go away and are part of the detoxification effects of vitamin D. In general your health will begin to improve following the phase of detoxification. Be aware that it is essential to keep an eye on levels of vitamin D and should consult a doctor when you're suffering from any disease or illness. The aim is to go from low amounts of vitamin D, to levels that are normal, and eventually maintain optimal levels for at minimum 90 days. It is important to up the volume of water you drink to assist in flushing out toxins from your body. Ensure that you perform moderate exercises at least four times per week. The entire process is efficient in not just detoxifying but also allowing anti-inflammatory benefits to be gradually absorbed into your body. Also, you will begin to notice weight loss since when you boost vitamin D levels, the hormones that are present in your body start to function effectively and help you cleanse and eliminate extra weight. Diet And Adding Vitamin D

One way to obtain vitamin D can be obtained is to gradually include foods that are rich in it. Then, you can examine your blood regularly to get the most accurate information. For instance, Joe has discovered that his blood test results show a low level of 23 ng/ml. He is now looking to start supplementing vitamin D2 into his the diet. However, he is worried about taking excessive vitamin D. So we just add seafood to the diet during his first week, and then will take another blood test: 29 ng/ml was the result. Bravo Joe! But he's aware that having higher amounts of vitamin D could assist in reducing or improving your chances of contracting an illness that is serious and maintain his health at higher levels. Joe decides to to consume the cod liver oil 3 times each week. He then sits in the sun in the noon hour for 20 minutes while taking the pants legs and shirt wrapped up. It's a huge change and then the following week Joe sees significant improvements of 48 ng/ml. Joe has the correct dosage and understands that it's crucial to track the effects of the supplementation in order that he is able to not only remain at an optimal level however, but keep improving his health and wellbeing. You can do the identical thing, and it's not too difficult. It just requires a commitment to regular blood tests, and adjustments of your exercise and diet. Keep your Vitamin D Naturally

Being able to maintain vitamin D naturally implies that it's not required to take supplements orally, but you can include more nutrients in your diet and increase Sun exposure. Most people's solution to lower levels in vitamin D are to go out and then begin taking supplements. But with fat-soluble vitamins, it is important to be aware, particularly with vitamin D which also functions as an hormone. There is no need for supplements, but rather to enhance your Sun exposure and the food items that we've suggested be added to your diet. Your body is far better equipped to manage naturally-sourced Vitamin D sources, and thus you are less likely to get a high. Also, you should think about the importance of regularly scheduled testing and monitoring your blood levels as well as talking to with a doctor because they could know things about your health that you haven't considered and that vitamin D might influence. For instance, if you suffer from tuberculosis, and taking vitamin D supplements could damage your health. For the normal person, even those suffering from a disease such as cancer or diabetes taking vitamin D supplements is vital since it will help maintain your well-being.

Chapter 6: "Definition Of Nutrients"

I believe that the best gift you can offer your family and friends is a healthy and happy you."

Joyce Meyer

We hear a lot regarding nutrition, and the importance of eating "nutrient rich" foods. What exactly is the definition of a nutritional element? What is its significance in our health? What are the tasks it plays in our bodies? In simple terms it is believed to be a part of the food items that living creatures require to survive and for growth reasons. Nutrients can be classified into two types:

Macronutrients They are the big players that provide the body with energy to perform the different metabolic functions. The body needs these nutrients in large amounts.

Micronutrients: Although not essential but they do give the body cofactors that assist in the working of metabolic processes. The need for these nutrients is not as high and they should be consumed in limited amounts. Both macronutrients and micronutrients are easily found in the world. They serve a multitude of roles to play within the body. They give the body energy, aid in the regulation of the bodily functions and assist in the development of new tissues and repair damaged ones. Animals and plants have various methods to absorb nutrition from the surrounding. Plants take in the nutrients from soil through their roots, while leaves absorb elements from the air. Animals have digestive systems that break down the food consumed and extracts macronutrients as well as micronutrients out of it. The macronutrients then are utilized to boost energy levels, while micronutrients help in the execution of various metabolic functions within the body.

Organic Nutrients: Proteins vitamins, carbohydrates, and fats

Inorganic Nutrients: Water oxygen, and mineral dietary sources.

That's the basic definition of the term "nutrient. Every product we consume contains some or all of the nutrients in it, with some being more than others. In order to keep our bodies healthy, it is essential to eat various nutrient-rich food items to ensure that the body gets all the necessary nutrients to perform metabolic functions. If you only eat unhealthy food items like French fries, the only thing you are getting is sugars, carbs, and sodium. This means that your body receives energy from food, but since junk food isn't rich in micronutrients the body can't complete metabolic tasks and that energy is being wasted. Recently, scientists recognized that if you meet the needs of both macronutrients and micronutrients, it doesn't necessarily mean one will live a healthy and happy life. This is evident by the rising number of various diseases that are prevalent in west. The proportion of people suffering from heart disease or cancer as well as weight gain is high these countries.

The reason is the rising amount of junk food that is incorporated into people's diets as well as the decreasing amount of physical activities. A balanced, healthy diet are always followed by some type of physical exercise to ensure you stay well and free of disease for the rest of your all of.

Chapter 7: Most Important Nutrients

"Health isn't valued until the time of illness."

Thomas F.

All nutrients are essential However, certain nutrients are more essential than other. The majority of people take in the proper quantity of nutrients just by chance however, they aren't aware of the exact proportion of nutrients required to develop. On a regular basis everyone consumes or loses a certain amount of nutrients when performing different tasks. In the event of an insufficient supply of a specific nutritional element in the body, the tissues of the body utilize the stored nutrients to satisfy the requirements. However, if the proper nutrients aren't stored and consumed in the body, it will result in an insufficient supply of nutrients that can cause a deficit.

As we have mentioned, some nutrients play a greater role in the body. Here are some nutrients that play an significant role in the body:

1. Proteins

The word comes from the Greek word that means being the one who holds the top spot. Proteins are the basis for the development of an organism. Proteins are composed of amino acids. They are often referred to as the primary building components of the human body. Protein is mostly found in butter, milk cereals, bread, bread and even meat. The people who are vegetarians consume proteins from fruits, legumes and vegetables as well as other dairy products. Vegans mostly get their protein from soy-based products.

2. Fats

The primary characteristic in fat is they're not liquid in water, however they dissolve in an organic compound called Acetone. The texture of fats is greasy and it is non-volatile. Fats are essential for performing metabolic and structural functions within the body.

Health experts have described fats in two ways, i.e. visible and invisibly. The visible fats include those that are visible to our naked eyes. They include butter, olive oil cheese, sunflower spread, as well as the fat contained that are found within meat chunks. The invisible fats comprise items such as junk food, pastries egg yolks and so on. In these cases, you can't see the fat content of the item.

3. Carbohydrates

Carbohydrates comprise the group of compounds that are typically present in both animals and plants. Although they aren't an essential food source but they are considered vital since they are the primary sources of energy for our bodies. Carbohydrates can be found in a wide range of food items like cereals, vegetables and pulses, dairy products as well as other foods. Most commonly, carbohydrates are present in processed food items. (d) Vitamins Vitamins are considered organic compounds that play an essential role in the body's metabolic processes. Vitamins may be water soluble or fat soluble according to their chemical composition. There are 14 vitamins that are known and some of the richest food sources for these nutrients include lean meats, dairy products as well as green leafy vegetables. fruits that are orange and yellow, as well as vegetables.

Chapter 8: Vitamin D

When wealth is lost, no thing is lost. However, when the health of a person is diminished, something gets lost. If the character of a person is destroyed, everything will be lost."

B. Graham

The first research are based in Vitamin D started from the condition of rickets. Rickets is a bone disorder that is typically seen in infants and the early years of the child's life. In 1919 the famous Sir Edward Mellanby proved that the illness is due to the deficiency of nutrition and also demonstrated that the condition was curable by the use of sunlight. In the following few years, various researchers, through the use of various research and experiments conducted research on the effects of UV radiation on children with rickets. They discovered that the nutrients derived from sunlight had a huge effect on children suffering from rickets. Vitamin D is believed as a subset of secosteroids, which are fat-soluble in the natural world. Secosteroids from this group aid the intestine in absorption of magnesium and iron, as well as zinc, calcium and the phosphate.

For humans as far as they are concerned the Cholecalciferol (vitamin D3) and ergocalciferol (vitamin D2) are extremely vital for development and growth goals. The body can't make these substances internally, so it is essential to attempt to incorporate vitamin D into our diets in addition to exposure to sunlight to create vitamin D in our bodies.

Different types of Vitamin D

There are a variety of vitamin D, based on the chemical makeup. The two most popular varieties of vitamin D are ergocalciferol (vitamin D2) and the cholecalciferol (vitamin D3).

Pure vitamin D with no subscript is either ergocalciferol , cholecalciferol, or even both. Vitamin D3 along with Vitamin D2 in combination are referred to as calciferol. The chemical structure of vitamin D2 was identified along with the structural structure that vitamin D3 was discovered in 1935 following investigating the effect of 7 dehydrocholestrol's effects on UV Rays.

The various types of vitamin D can be chemically identified as secosteroids. Secosteroids are thought to be steroids with the broken bond of steroid inside their rings. The vitamin is classified into three kinds according to their chemical composition

1. Vitamin DI

2. Vitamin D.

3. Vitamin D3

4. Vitamin D4

5. Vitamin D5

Chapter 9: Factors That Influence The Production Of Vitamin D

The excitement of vitamins metabolism, and nutrition permeated the atmosphere."

Paul D. Boyer

Many biological influences can influence the production and production of Vitamin D3 in the body. The most significant of these are ageing, fashion of clothes, exposure to the sun, the excessive use of sunscreen lotions diverse types of pollution and the changing seasons. In all the possible reasons the degree of pigmentation and ageing is the most significant one.

1. Pigmentation of the Skin

A lesser amount of solar radiation as well as skin pigmentation are two factors that impact your production Vitamin D3. This is because of melanin's presence, which combats the dehydrocholesterol 7 and blocks the absorption of ultra-violate radiations that are necessary for vitamin D3 metabolism in the body.

2. Aging

As you age the skin begins to thin. The process starts when you reach the age of 20. The level of the seven-dehydrocholesterol keeps on increasing with your growing age, but the production of vitamin D3 does not increase due to the thinning skin. Young adults can produce around three times more vitamin D than their elders. As time goes by your skin's thickness is declining, leading to lower production of vitamin D.

Chapter 10: Hidden Benefits Of Vitamin D

To keep your body healthy is a requirement... or else we are unable to keep our mind healthy as well as clear."

Buddha

Vitamin D is required for human health for many different functions. One of the most significant actions that requires vitamin D is the growth of bones. Vitamin D assists calcium to be absorbed by the body of all living thing, and, as we all know, calcium is vital to bone growth within the body. Additionally it is useful in the development and growth of heart muscles and fat tissues as well as brain cells. Vitamin D regulates various cells' development and growth within the body. That is the reason it is a vital nutritional element for our body. Furthermore it is also helpful in the control of metabolic processes as well as the immune functions that take place within the body. In the past few years, vitamin D has been gaining recognition. Vitamin D has led experts to engage in a never-ending discussion.

Certain studies suggest that vitamin D alone doesn't have an effect specifically, however when it is connected to other processes, it can be extremely beneficial. However, studies have shown that blood vessels that contain vitamin D contain a high amount of toxins, which can cause various serious cardiovascular problems within the body. This could result in the premature death of a person.

Vitamin D to help lose weight

It is health that is real wealth, not bits of silver and gold."

Gandhi

Researchers believe that vitamin D is loaded with benefits for humans. It may have the solutions to many of the most talked about and controversial research. In the past, it was believed that vitamin D might help fight heart disease, cancer and may even assist with weight reduction. There was no proof that vitamin D can aid in weight loss until a group of scientists from the Fred Hutchinson Cancer Research Center was studying several overweight women with a insufficient levels in vitamin D. They found that these women lost weight over the course of 12 months. The women were taking constant, and a set quantity in vitamin D supplementation. Additionally they followed an exercise program that was daily. Researchers also noticed that the women who were in the middle of being overweight were slimmer. The weight loss for both types of groups was quite normal. When the women were compared to women who were following strict diets The results were identical. The researchers concluded their research with the belief that vitamin D can aid in treating health issues such as obesity.

The Relationship Between Calcium and Vitamin D

To live an active and healthy life it is essential to have solid and sturdy bones. Calcium is among the minerals that are vital to the existence of living organisms. Together calcium and vitamin D make up the main loop that helps living things last for a long time. Calcium is among the minerals that help keep our bones in good health. However, it is not the only one however, it is also involved in the clotting process of blood and transmits signals to the nerves leading to the contraction of muscles. When we look at the proportion of calcium present in the human body living beings, around 90% of it is found in bones as well as the teeth. It's also found in hair, skin and nails, as well as in urine or even sweat. So, each day we shed a little bit of calcium in our bodies and therefore, it is required to be replenished on a regular basis.

1. Calcium

The Bone The Body Bones contain a separate compartment for fluids, that is isolated from other areas. The bone's compartment is a space that is filled with the fluid, which is located between the thin skin linings that surround the cells as well as the matrix bone. Thus, it is located in close contact with bones.

The ratio of calcium in bone fluid is typically around one third higher than other fluids, such as within extracellular fluid. There are tiny lining cells that line the outside of the bone, as well as in the fluid. These tiny cells have open channels that allow for calcium to flow into the bone's fluid. The flow of the fluid to the upward direction requires the process of transportation that will move it through the lining of cells.

2. Vitamin D and bones

It has been proven it is true that vitamin D is essential for smooth and normal development of bones. It is also helpful in the process of mineralization which results in the remodelling of bones. Researchers have also suggested that the importance for vitamin D during the growth of bone is crucial because it assists in the passage of calcium from one stage to another. It assists calcium to absorb into the various bone sections. This whole process is supported by the higher absorption rate of minerals within the digestive tract.

Affordable sources of Vitamin D

Vitamin D isn't often found in food. It is possible that the skin absorbs a most of the vitamin from the sun. In terms of foods we eat, the liver oils from fish as well as fatty fishes like tuna, pilchards and herring are just a few of the of foods that are rich in vitamin D. In addition to fishes, vitamin D is also present in the liver of mammals as well as dairy products like drinks made from milk, however the amount of vitamin D is not enough. Food items like fruits, vegetables and cereals contain no Vitamin D. That's the reason the majority of vegetarians and vegans are at chance of developing a vitamin D deficit and should spend lots of time in the sun, or in extreme instances you should use vitamins D supplements.

Chapter 11: Vitamin D Deficiency

As previously mentioned the most important elements that influence the creation of Vitamin D in the body are darker skin tones, deficiency of sunlight breastfeeding, and without supplements. When there is vitamin D deficiency, manufacturing of calcium-binding protein is reduced. So, when calcium present in the body is not accompanied by being bound by this protein it travels through the body without being absorption. Due to the lack of vitamin D, teenagers aren't likely to live a long and well-balanced life and are likely to suffer from huge amounts from calcium deficiency. The increase in deficiency can cause the child develop other chronic illnesses.

1. Osteomalacia

If you're too old, the body will require the same amount of Vitamin D. As you age and the body's requirement for Vitamin D remains the same however, the skin becomes thin and as a result of long-term aging, the skin becomes in no position to make the vitamin. The result is painful, numbness throughout the night and, at times, swelling. Due to the lack in Vitamin D, the bones become fragile and soft and in some cases they become damaged. (1) Rickets Rickets is the most popular and often diagnosed disease in children. The proportion of children affected by the disease is greater in less developed and developed nations. Tibet, Mongolia and Netherlands are just a few of countries with lots of children who suffer from rickets. Even in developed nations like the United States of America, there are many instances of the illness being reported. The majority of kids that suffer from the disease, have dark skin. The percentage of girls who suffer from rickets is greater than the boys. To prevent the spread of the disease the government of America provides a number of injections or drugs to provide the body with vitamin as well as aid in the prevention and treatment of the condition. When the disease is present the bones of the sufferer become weak. The reason for this is that the bones aren't getting the calcium they require to keep their strength. To help support their whole body they are able to bend a bit and walk, ruining their posture for the rest of their lives.

2. Osteoporosis

The human body doesn't get enough of vitamin D, either from their diet or sunlight, they develop weak bones. This is because vitamin D's main role in the absorption and utilization of calcium by the body and the transportation of calcium within the body. It also aids bones soak up the calcium and gain the strength and mass. Osteoporosis literally translates to "porous bone" to Greek. The density and the weight of bones diminish and increase the likelihood of sustaining fractures. In this condition, the bone mineral density (BMD) is reduced, resulting in a higher incidence of falls and breaking of bones among those who suffer from it. The condition is typically observed in women, and female patients surpass male patients by a percentage.

3. Elders

As we've already mentioned in the past, as we getting older Vitamin D production is decreasing. As a person reaches their old age and their body's parts aren't functioning correctly. That is, internal organs such as liver, kidney and skin produce little vitamin D. It isn't sufficient for proper functioning of the body in its entirety. In the end, many times seniors spend a significant portion of their time at their home. Their bodies are unable to taking in some Vitamin D that is absorbed from sunlight. Even when they leave from their houses wearing layers of clothing, which it becomes impossible for UV rays from the sun to come into contact with the skin. All these things affect the bones of their bodies which makes them more fragile and more supple to their body's structure.

Infertility

The management of fertility is among of the most important responsibilities in adulthood."

G. Greer

4. Female

The proportion of infertility ranges between percent and percent in 30-40% of cases when one spouse suffers from infertility. The remaining portion of the rate, i.e. 20-40%, aren't aware of the root cause, and there are couples where both couples are infertile. After a number of studies, and studies, experts have been able to demonstrate that changes in the seasons and climate can affect quality of the sperm as well as the ratio of ovulation and the ovulation ratio. In numerous studies, women received different forms of vitamin D3 together with a certain quantity of calcium and the mineral phosphorus. After a few months women who were not capable of conceiving earlier were able to get an ovulation that was successful and have an ovulated and healthy and fertile litter. Through the above research researchers discovered the fact that Vitamin D alone does not cause infertility. But, it's associated with calcium and the phosphorus. Additionally they found that climate and temperature can play an important role.

5. Male

In the previous case we've previously talked about the rate of infertility among one of the couples. A variety of studies in the past have proven that vitamin D an effect on men's reproductive systems in animals. In humans vitamin D functions as an substance that plays an important role in the mechanisms and the various functions that are related to men's reproductive systems as well as the whole process. It influences the various agents, including cholesterol efflux, protein, and cholesterol and calcium levels, and permits an independent and spontaneous movement that results in the longevity of the male sperm. Studies have shown that people who had Vitamin D deficiency had lower rate of sperm movements in comparison to those who have normal levels in Vitamin D.

Through years of study and research scientists have concluded that the declining ratio of testosterone in males is by a variety of factors and the low level in vitamin D could be just one of the causes. However, its impact on the infertility problem is much more prominent in females.

6. Insulin Secretion

Dihydroxyvitamin D3 is believed to be the ingredient that aids in the release of insulin. The results of studies showed that the alteration in the ratio of vitamin D, which is a protein found in the pancreas as well as other organs of the body may affect the whole process of the production of insulin.

Chapter 12: Overconsumption Vitamin D

Vitamins are an essential molecule found in the living organism. We are all aware of the role that vitamin D is involved in the absorption of calcium within the body as well as the transportation of calcium to different organs. In addition is the fact that it assists to absorb calcium into the bones. But, too much vitamin D are risky for all. We have learned the ways that vitamin D can help living creatures live a long and healthy life. We also discussed how a lack of vitamin D could lead to many different diseases that can be fatal in long-term.

The toxic effects of Vitamin D

Vitamin D can be extremely beneficial and essential to perform various functions within the body. However, the excess of it could cause a lot of problems for you. The fat-soluble vitamin can cause harm if you consume it in a large amounts. It is believed that the amount that is produced by our skin, and is consumed through food items is sufficient in order for the body's functions to work correctly and is the best amount of Vitamin D. In some instances those who are lacking in vitamin D consume various supplements to get a healthy level of Vitamin D in their bodies. However, they must keep an eye on one thing: supplements should not be administered to children. In the body, a young child can create their own vitamins in a natural method. Even adults are instructed to take the vitamin supplement in a specific ratio for a specific time.

The excess of Vitamin D could increase the amount of calcium present in blood. Blood that is contaminated with a high amount of calcium could cause the destruction of all soft tissues. This results in the formation of stones. These are then deposited inside the kidneys, as an attempt to release the hormone.

Chapter 13: Understanding Foundations Of Vitamin D

Vitamin D was associated with strong bones as early as the 19th century, when doctors realized that exposure to sunlight could help in the prevention of rickets which is a bone disease commonly seen in children. To treat the condition, using cod liver oil and taking a bath in the sun could help significantly. When milk was fortified using Vitamin D in the western world 100 years later the disease was almost completely eliminated. The more studies that were conducted on Vitamin D, the more it was discovered to be essential for general health, not only bone health. Actually, Vitamin D can help in the prevention and treatment of many serious health problems.

Vitamin D is an individual vitamin distinct from other vitamins our bodies require. To understand the ways it does amazing things, we must be aware of the nature of Vitamin D is. Let's take a look at the fundamentals that comprise Vitamin D.

What exactly is Vitamin D?

The most shocking thing regarding Vitamin D can be that it's not an actual vitamin. It's not really. Experts in medicine say they prefer to refer to it as a hormone because the body produces it by itself with the assistance of the sun. Numerous other vitamins, including zinc, calcium and potassium are also elements you can identify within the daily chart, and they need to be taken in.

When the skin is exposed to sunlight and Vitamin D is made and absorbed, it goes to the liver to process. If you ingest the Vitamin D supplement The Vitamin D is also delivered to your liver via the digestive tract. Doctors refer to the substance as converts in "calcidiol" also known as 25(OH) D. This word is used to describe the quantity of Vitamin D in blood, and is a reference to the serum.

This chemical is transported throughout the body, to various tissues. It regulates the amount of calcium that is found in bones and blood and, in this way, it helps all cells in our body interact. The kidneys convert to "activated Vitamin D," or calcitriol. It is then absorbed into the body to perform many other functions. Vitamin D can be described as a mighty vitamin because it is utilized by virtually every cell in the body.

Different types of Vitamin D The D2 type is different from the D3

Vitamin D exists in two forms: Vitamin D3 as well as Vitamin D2. Vitamin D3 is created by exposure to sunlight. It's more frequent that Vitamin D2.

Vitamin D2 is referred to as Ergocalciferol. It's not present by itself in nature. Instead, it is the result of irradiated fungal species. It can find in fortified food items including cereals, plants, food items and supplements. It is Vitamin D is suggested by medical professionals if there isn't Vitamin D3 in the market, or for vegetarians, however it is considered insufficient.

The body produces Vitamin D3, also known as Cholecalciferol from the sunlight. It's also present in certain fish. Vitamin D3 supplementation is usually made from the fats of sheep's wool or fish oil.

What is Vitamin D Effective for General Health?

Vitamin D helps improve the strength and health of bones. It also aids in increasing the efficiency of your muscles, heart, lungs and brain which can assist your body to fight many illnesses.

When it comes to bone development Calcium and phosphorus are crucial to bone strength and development. Vitamin D is essential to absorb these minerals. Foods contain sufficient or even excessive quantities in calcium as well as phosphorus however, without Vitamin D the body isn't capable of absorbing these minerals.

Vitamin D offers a variety of benefits throughout the body. It makes an important difference in the health of bones, blood and organs of the body. Vitamin D improves the performance of various functions within the body, including the treatment and prevention of:

Diabetes

Cancer

Skeletal disorders

Immune systems that are weak

Heart and circulatory function

Sleep disorders

Depression

Obesity

Chapter 14: Where To Find Your Vitamin D

Vitamin D is distinct in comparison to other vitamins due to the fact that the body is able to create it itself when you expose it to sunlight. If you're not able to enjoy the sun, you can still get Vitamin D by taking supplements. Vitamin D can be found in small amounts in handful of foods, such as oily fish, as well as in food items that have been supplemented, such as margarine, yogurt, milk and cereal.

Being exposed to moderate amounts of sunshine can aid in getting the everyday dose Vitamin D but it may not suffice. This is particularly true in the event that you're not able to sit for extended time in the sun or, due to the weather that you don't have sunlight whatsoever. Contrary to other vitamins, Vitamin D is not able to take in enough food to meet the amount recommended by Vitamin D.

Vitamin D that sunlight produces is derived from UVB (UVB) Rays. The amount your body produces is contingent on a variety of factors, including:

What time of the day you're exposed to sun? The most effective sun's rays are for Vitamin D absorption is around midday. The early morning and late afternoon sunlight is not enough because the atmospheric blockage blocks the important UVB radiations during the time.

The country in which you reside The closer the place that you reside in is the equator the more convenient you can get your skin's absorption of Vitamin D. Regions that are further away from the equator will experience extreme weather patternsthat impact the amount of sunlight that can be absorbed.

Your skin's color - Those with pale skins do not have to spend a lot of time in the sun to get Vitamin D absorption. This contrasts to those with darker skin.

The amount you exercise Research has revealed that those who regularly exercise are carrying more than 25 (OH) D levels in their blood. It is particularly interesting that this appears to be the case regardless of whether the individual is working out outside.

Vitamin D and Sun Exposure

An excellent guideline for knowing when you've been exposed enough is to stay out in sun about half the amount of time that you must be until you get sunburn. Fair skinned people can safely be exposed to the sun to the sun for about 10 minutes, while those with darker skin tone might require two hours of exposure to the sun. During this period, your body will produce anywhere between 10,000 to 25,000 IU of Vitamin D.

It is essential for your skin to be exposed to absorb some Vitamin D through the sun's radiation. Therefore, being outside in sun with pants and a long-sleeved t-shirt can limit the amount of Vitamin D that your body is able to absorb. Ideally, any surface, like the back of your body, would be ideal. It's not enough to obtain enough Vitamin D through just making sure you expose your arms and face.

A lot of sun exposure but it can result in sunburn. The sunburns could result in skin cancer. Applying sunblock is a good option to shield your skin from UV rays that cause harm However, it also blocks beneficial ones. Actually, sunscreens can reduce Vitamin D absorbtion by as much as 95 percent. The apparently healthy habit of applying sunblock whenever you are in the sun is an important cause of Vitamin D deficiencies. It is a in a thin line of absorbing enough sunlight to produce Vitamin D however, not to the point of burn.

Other variables influence the amount of Vitamin D that your body is able to produce. One of them is the age. The older you get the more difficult it will be for your skin to make Vitamin D. Therefore, older people are advised to consume more Vitamin D supplements.

When it's cloudy, the skin's production of Vitamin D which is also the case if you reside in an area with a lot of pollution from the air. This is due to the fact that sunlight's rays are prevented from reaching the skin. Additionally, UVB radiations cannot penetrate glass, so when you're driving with your windows closed on a day that is sunny the skin won't be able to create Vitamin D.

Tanning beds are an effective method to get your daily dose of vitamin D if you use them appropriately. Limit your time to a short amount of time, and ensure that it's a low-pressure bed that is well-lit with plenty of UVB light.

Vitamin D in food

The body produces it own Vitamin D through absorbing sunlight's rays. Supplements are also a major factor. But, there are foods that have small amounts in Vitamin D as well.

Vitamin D is found in the cod liver oil however, it is also Vitamin A and Vitamin A in large quantities. Since both nutrients are fat-soluble and fat soluble, your body could have a difficult time absorbing the vitamin. Additionally, since the composition in cod liver oil may differ widely depending on the person who made it, doctors are now hesitant about suggesting it as the principal source of Vitamin D. Other foods that are rich in Vitamin D include fatty fish such as mackerel and salmon cereals with fortified ingredients eggs, yolks of eggs along with fortified milk, beef liver as well as infant formula.

When you've figured out your daily recommended intake then you'll be able to understand why people don't get all of their Vitamin D through food by itself. For instance, a tablespoon of oil from cod liver has 1260IU of Vitamin D. It's true that a 3.5 1 ounce portion of salmon cooked in a pan contains 360 IU vitamin D. The equivalent amount of swordfish contains more, 566 IU. That's almost a whole day's worth of Vitamin D for adults. Canned tuna contains an average of 154 IU for 3 ounces. And if you like Sardines, they're a good source of 46 IU. Fortified milk has the equivalent of 98 IU of Vitamin D for each cup. an entire egg has 20 IU, while fortified cereals contain 40 IU per each cup. The yogurt that is enhanced can contain more than 127 IU in a cup. Beef kidneys and beef livers are a good source of 40 IU per 3 ounces, however other red meats aren't as rich in.

Adults need at least 600 mg of Vitamin D every daily. You could get it through eating cereal with milk for breakfast, and a cup of yogurt that is fortified to eat lunch, and salmon for dinner as well as plenty of fruit and vegetables, and maybe whole grains to help balance the meals. You can substitute meat or chicken for dinnerand you'll notice that your Vitamin D intake is reduced to half.

Chapter 15: Breaking Down Vitamin D Deficiency

I had the pleasure of meeting a woman known as Marianne within an Vitamin D discussion group, and I'd like to tell this story. Marianne's legs were always hurting. Pain medication available over the counter helped a only a little, but the narcotic pain medication caused her to be nauseated. The doctor could not provide any reason for her constant painor the constant tiredness she was experiencing. He suggested practicing yoga and meditation to manage the "stress" that she was experiencing in her daily life. The administrator of forty-four as well as mother to three experienced plenty of stress However, she recognized that there was something else going on. Her symptoms could be caused by the weight she put on over time or that perimenopausal symptoms were getting more severe and she was scared that she was never going to improve. Jeff her husband believed she was within her brain.

A friend finally encouraged her to visit an additional doctor who requested a variety of tests. One of them was checking for Vitamin D. The levels of Marianne's were low. The doctor prescribed the highest dose of supplements. After several months, she started to feel more normal.

Marianne's tale is very extreme yet everyday people all around the world complain to their doctors regarding muscle pain, fatigue chronic illness, depression and much more. The doctors are beginning to monitor Vitamin D levels frequently. A study from 2009 that was published in The Scientific American suggests that 75 percent of the US population is not getting enough Vitamin D. The Center for Disease Control and Prevention estimates that the figure can rise to 90% when you're African American. The good news is that the problem is expected to be brought under control over the next years as doctors begin to link daily vitamin D supplements to reducing or even curing a range of ailments.

The body suffers from an Vitamin D deficiency if it isn't getting enough Vitamin D for normal functioning. If a child suffers from severe

Vitamin D deficiency, they are thought to suffer from Rickets. They might appear bow-legged and, if young, they may have difficulties standing or moving frequently. Sometimes, the condition can be misinterpreted as child abuse due to the bones snap easily.

If an adult suffers from a significant Vitamin D deficiency, the disease is called osteomalacia. The deficiency could cause fragile, soft, and bone fragments that could cause fractures of bone due to falls or loss of balance.

Vitamin D Deficiency is linked to serious health problems and some of them can be considered to be terminal. It can lead to cancers and high blood pressure. asthma, type II diabetes and type I diabetes. Multiple sclerosis and Alzheimer's. Conditions that affect muscles can also arise because of Vitamin D deficiencies.

The causes and symptoms for Vitamin D Deficiency

Most likely triggers for Vitamin D deficiency are:

The body isn't exposed to enough sun. The reason is that most people spend a lot of their time inside. Another factor can be the usage of sunscreens which prevents the skin from absorption UVB radiation.

Many people do not supplement adequately. Vitamin D is present in small amounts in foods and almost all people have to supplement, especially during the winter months. If you're deficient in D3, the quantity that is found in a variety of multivitamins may not be enough.

Certain people are more prone to Vitamin D deficiencies than others. They are those with darker skintones, especially those with black skin. The higher the amount of melanin within the skin the more difficult it is to absorb sunlight's ultraviolet rays. It's been discovered that those with dark skin can be exposed to 25 times more than those who are fair.

People who work in indoors, in hospitals, tunnels or during the night are also often victims since they are less likely to be able to take advantage of the sun's rays. Additionally, those who are covered often, especially in areas with colder temperatures and less hours of sun exposure every day. People who are older and have fragile skin might not produce sufficient Vitamin D. Infants who exclusively breast milk or whose mothers do not consume a supplement, or who do not get exposure to sunlight and sun, are more likely to have deficiencies. The obese or pregnant women may also be at risk since they require higher than normal dosages.

There are a variety of signs that can be observed to detect a serious Vitamin D deficit. It is crucial to remember that these signs are obscure and, in some instances it is possible that no symptoms are evident at all.

The symptoms are:

Tiredness

The body is aching and painful throughout the body

It feels as if it is inside the bones

General weakness of the body

It is difficult to move around and perform physical tasks

Infections that are frequent.

To see if you've got enough Vitamin D within your body, your doctor will perform the blood test to measure the 25(OH) D levels.

Effects of Taking too much Vitamin D

In excess of a positive thing could turn out to be extremely negative. If you consume Vitamin D supplements in excess your body could be left with excessive levels of calcium in your blood. This causes the condition called hypercalcemia. The symptoms are:

Feelings of confusion

Exhaustion

The thirst and illness of the body

A loss of appetite

Continuous passage of urine

Muscle weakness and abdominal pain

To determine whether you've consumed a lot in Vitamin D in your supplements The doctor will need to perform an analysis of your blood.

Vitamin D toxicities are often referred to as Hypervitaminosis D and could be a risky health condition. It's often caused by taking massive amounts of Vitamin supplements, not due to excessive exposure to sunlight or through diet. The body is able to regulate the amount Vitamin D it makes due to sun exposure. Foods don't contain sufficient Vitamin D to create this kind of risk (though eating a lot of foods high in D may cause other issues).

Vitamin D toxicity can cause calcium accumulation in the body, leading to nausea, loss of appetite and other signs of hypercalcemia. The toxicity levels are attained when more than 10,000 IU of Vitamin D is consumed each daily for many months.

There are many options for treatment. First, quit the intake of Vitamin D in excess. Doctors might also prescribe bisphosphonates or corticosteroids and may recommend you reduce the calcium content in your diet.

There are long-term issues which could arise because of hypervitaminosis D if it's neglected. They are mostly related with kidneys and can are kidney-related and include damage, stones as well as kidney dysfunction. There could also be a loss of bone that causes calcium calcification in the arteries and an increase in blood calcium levels that could trigger abdominal heart rhythms.

In addition to an Blood test, however, you might have been diagnosed with Vitamin D toxicities following an urine test which looks for calcium levels that are excessive or bone x-rays in search of significant bone loss.

The Serum and Vitamin D Vitamin D Levels and Serum Levels Understanding the Lab Test Results

There is a agreement that the serum levels are the most crucial aspect to keep in mind in determining the concentrations of Vitamin D within the body. This is what the number 25 (OH) D is. How these levels are perceived aren't the same as being universally accepted However, the most popular levels are:

(OH) Level (OH) D

Deficient < 50 ng/ ml

Ideal 50 - 70 ng/ml

Treats heart disease and cancer 70-100 mg/ml

Exceeding 100 ng/ml

Chapter 16: What You Have To Learn About Vitamin D Supplements

It could be a struggle to get enough time every day outside in the sun to achieve the daily recommended amount of Vitamin D. However, supplements are available to assist your body obtain the nutrients it requires.

There are two types of Vitamin D supplements. The most popular one can be Vitamin D3. It's typically offered as capsules or tablets, but it can also be found in creams for skin. These supplements are made from the wool fat or fish oil, and are not vegan-friendly. Vitamin D3 is akin to the function that is Vitamin D that is created by sunlight.

Vitamin D2 supplements are made from plants and are not advised, except for vegetarians. Vitamin D3 is transformed faster in the body, and can be converted up to 500% more quickly as Vitamin D2. Vitamin D2 has also been believed to have a much shorter shelf time. Another issue with Vitamin D2 is that its compounds are not well-integrated with proteins, which results in its being less efficient in comparison to Vitamin D3.

Vitamin D supplements are available in a variety of strengths, with the majority being 10,000 IU or 5,000 IU per unit. If you suffer from serious deficiencies, a physician may recommend the 500,00 IU dose to take each week or once solely to stay clear of Vitamin D toxicities.

Vitamin D supplements can be found in an oil drop emulsified with oil as well as chewable tablets or capsule, or as a cream applied to the skin. There are some scientists who think it is possible that Vitamin D supplements are better taken in the form of chewing and moving through the tongue.

Vitamin D is a Vitamin D supplement is prescribed by a physician however, many forms are available to purchase on the internet. It is crucial to verify for the correct dosage when buying these vitamins over market. They are Vitamin D2 and Vitamin D3 supplements typically have similar in cost. There are Vitamin

D3 supplements that also contain calcium and are in the market. They are typically prescribed to patients with bone disorders who require calcium and make sure that calcium is absorbed in the right amount.

To get the most effective absorption results, Vitamin D supplements should be taken in conjunction with meals that contain fat. If one consumes an Vitamin D supplement with no food then the standard amount for Vitamin D absorption drops by 32 percent. The fats that are transported with the supplement implies that Vitamin D does not have to travel through the body to locate fat under the skin.

Vitamin D supplements can interact with certain medications , and result in their ineffectiveness. This is especially true for steroid medicines such as Prednisone that can interfere with Vitamin D metabolism. Before taking the choice to purchase prescription Vitamin D, they should talk to their doctor, especially in the case of other medication.

Furthermore some weight loss medications and seizure medication can cause problems with calcium absorption as well as Vitamin D metabolism. Certain drugs that are used to reduce cholesterol are believed to raise levels of Vitamin D levels within the body. This is a great idea, but it could be cause harm if the supplement is being consumed simultaneously.

Chapter 17: Recommendations For Vitamin D Consumption

In the world, many organizations around the world will give their own guidelines on the amount of Vitamin D is needed for every day. A few common numbers for recommended minimum daily intakes include:

Age-Recommended Daily Intake

Infants 400 IU

Children 400 IU

Adults 600 Inj.

Seniors 800 IU

Between adults and infants The dosage of this dose supports the idea that the larger and heavier you are the higher the amount of Vitamin D you require in order to make sure that the body will perform at its peak. Seniors require more Vitamin D because their thin skin makes it difficult for sunlight's rays.

There are limits to these guidelines, particularly since certain supplements are not readily available in smaller amounts. This means that one can:

Age-Maximum Daily Intake

Infants 1000- 1500 IU

Children 2500 - 3000 IU

Adults 4000 I.U.

The reason it is crucial to not consume a large volume of Vitamin D is due to the fact that it is fat-soluble. This means that any excess amount is kept in the fat cells and will accumulate in your body as time passes. The maximum limit to adults of 4000IU a day, however that's considering that you are in the sunlight. If you don't spend much time outdoors Some believe that you could take as much as 10,000 IU per day, but it is recommended to consult an expert. Anything higher than this isn't considered to be safe or healthy. Repetition in Vitamin D overconsumption can lead to Vitamin D toxicity.

Vitamin D supplementation is simply supplements. It is important to spend as long outside in sunlight as feasible and secure. The sun's rays is believed to be responsible for 10,000 to 25,000 IU in Vitamin D being produced in the course of a single day. The body can manage Vitamin D from the sun that eliminates the problem of excessive levels if the sun is used as an energy source.

Chapter 18: Vitamin D And Diabetes

Vitamin D has been able to acquire a variety of names over the years and has been dubbed the sunshine vitamin' as well as the'miracle vitamin'. Researchers have discovered the fact that this Vitamin is great for the immune system. Some individuals have gone as far as to say that a balanced dosage of Vitamin D is better than any other vaccine.

This section will discuss the connection with Vitamin D and certain diseases and explains why Vitamin D is an ideal option for overall well-being and health.

Vitamin D and Type I Diabetes

It is an autoimmune disorder that occurs when the immune system targets beta cells, which are the pancreas' cells which help the body make the hormone known as insulin. Insulin aids in controlling glucose levels, and converts food into energy that the body to utilize.

There is a connection in the relationship between diabetes type I and Vitamin D. In essence, it was discovered that people who had a inadequate Vitamin D intake during the first year of their lives were more likely to develop type I diabetes as they became older. Pregnant women who lack Vitamin D can also affect their children, who could become diabetics of type I as they grow older.

In the treatment of type I diabetes it is recommended to take Vitamin D supplements could help increase insulin sensitivity and assist the blood in regulating sugar levels. While the research regarding the efficacy on the effectiveness of Vitamin D to treat type I diabetes isn't conclusive however, it's worthwhile to try it out in order to improve your health.

Vitamin D can't replace medications for type I diabetes.

Vitamin D and Type II Diabetes

The condition is known as Type II Diabetes. It's which causes the body to experience difficulties in managing sugar in a proper way. It's typically seen in people who are older and can last throughout life.

If the condition isn't properly treated, an individual may suffer from skin problems or high blood pressure, as well as issues with vision. The condition begins as mild, but it gets more severe with time. In the final stages of the disease organ malfunction, infections of the fingers and toes that can lead to amputation, as well as urinary tract problems can develop.

While research on the connection between Vitamin D and type II diabetes isn't conclusive, there is a study that has shown that those who are younger and have higher amounts of Vitamin D in their systems are less likely to develop Type II Diabetes later on in life. This was discovered when the people who had these levels were directly compared to people who had lower levels Vitamin D.

It is recommended to take an Vitamin D supplement for those suffering from type II Diabetes has been proven to ease the symptoms. It is not Vitamin D on its own an effective treatment for diabetes, but it can be a helpful aid.

In the treatment of type II diabetes Vitamin D is known to aid in turning on receptors in beta cells of the pancreas that are not functioning properly. This assists to produce insulin. Vitamin D is also helpful in controlling calcium. This is important since calcium plays an important role in regulating the release insulin, which could influence beta cell function.

Chapter 19: Vitamin D And Cancer

There are many cancers that impact the body. These cancers are able to attack any type of cell. They vary in the degree of attack and where they are located however, they do have one thing they all have in common: If ignored they could cause death before their time.

Vitamin D has been proven to be a great aid to patients suffering from cancer, since it can help ease the symptoms. Vitamin D can help reduce depression, and may even assist cancer patients fight it when coupled in conjunction with treatment options. This chapter will examine three cancers that are common and describe the ways these cancers are positively affected due to Vitamin D.

Vitamin D and Colorectal Cancer

If a set of cancerous cells decide to develop in the colon or rectum and form a malignant tumor, it is known as colorectal cancer. To determine the level of this disease, one must evaluate how large the cancer and whether or not it has spread to other areas within the human body.

The study of this kind of cancer, as well as Vitamin D has unearthed that colorectal cancer patients are more likely to suffer from low levels of Vitamin D. In fact those who have greater levels of Vitamin D are less likely to develop cancer of the colorectal. If you have had this type of cancer by increasing the Vitamin D levels could result in an improved outcome overall and reduce the risk of dying due to cancer.

Vitamin D assists in protecting against cancer of the colon because it contains receptors located on the cell's surface, which is where chemical signals can be received. These receptors aid the cell function in a specific manner. Vitamin D is able to bind these receptors, which causes the signals for division or death so that they do not be able to reach the cell, and prevent the spread of the body.

The research conducted is mostly observational, and shouldn't be relied upon completely particularly if it is viewed as a replacement for medication.

Vitamin D is also known as Breast Cancer

The cause of breast cancer lies in cancerous tumors in and around the breasts which cause an aggressive tumor.

Women who have breast cancer have been identified to have lower levels Vitamin D in their bodies. The risk for developing cancer in the breast reduces little for women with greater levels of Vitamin D. Women already suffering from breast cancer increasing their recommended daily doses of Vitamin D has shown that tumors in their bodies can shrink and their odds of being diagnosed with breast cancer are lower.

Vitamin D cannot be used as a cure for breast cancer, but it could help in getting more healthy. It is essential not to consume a dose over the upper limit of the daily recommended intake. It is also crucial not to think of the consumption of Vitamin D as a replacement for other treatments.

Vitamin D helps to treat breast cancer the exact manner like it works with colorectal cancer. Vitamin D binds receptors that allow the chemical signal to be processed.

Vitamin D is also known as Prostate Cancer

Prostate cancer is a condition that occurs in the prostate gland, located in a gland which is about one-quarter of the size as walnuts become abnormally large, leading to lumps of tissue called tumors that form. This type of cancer is more prevalent among older males.

Vitamin D was proven to be linked to prostate cancer. Men who have low amounts of Vitamin D are more susceptible to developing this cancer. People who are diagnosed with this cancer however maintain healthy levels of Vitamin D will be less likely to succumb to the cancer or suffer an especially aggressive form.

As with other types of cancer, Vitamin D attaches itself to receptors on cells, which results in slow or even stopped growth and death, or a reduced growth of cancerous cells.

The research is ongoing regarding the effectiveness on the effectiveness of Vitamin D and prostate cancer treatment. Vitamin D is not a viable option as a substitute for treatment.

Chapter 20: Vitamin D And Other Conditions

Alongside diabetes and cancer, Vitamin D is of tremendous aid to the body when fighting a variety of other ailments. These illnesses include those that are caused by problems with muscles, as well as those that impact bone.

To better understand the impact on the effect that Vitamin D has on these illnesses, this chapter provides more details on these aspects.

Vitamin D as well as Skeletal Conditions

The most serious diseases that affect the bones are directly connected to the calcium level and Vitamin D. If you are taking any dose of calcium that is to be absorbed by bones, it's essential to supplement it along with Vitamin D. It is due to the fact that Vitamin D aids in calcium absorption, keeping blood calcium levels, as well as prevents level of calcium in the blood. Together with calcium Vitamin D aids in the prevention of osteoporosis and osteomalacia. osteopenia.

Seniors with skeletal ailments are more prone to suffering serious bone fractures in the event they fall. The consumption of Vitamin D can prevent the 5.6 percent rate of fractures which occur in people who are older due to falling. In addition, Vitamin D strengthen the bones as well, but it also has receptors in muscles that enhance the strength of muscles.

Strengthening muscles can help increase balance. Indeed, studies have shown that consuming 1000 IU daily of Vitamin D3 can decrease the chance of falling by as much as 26 percent. The skeletal diseases caused by a Vitamin D deficiency could also cause pain in the hips as well as knees. The problem can be addressed in time by increasing amount of Vitamin D ingested on a regular basis.

Vitamin D as well as the Immune System

Researchers conducting research on Vitamin D have discovered that Vitamin D plays a part to aid in the strengthening of our immune system. The only thing that remains to be found out is the amount of Vitamin D required to boost the immune system.

This Vitamin is commonly referred to as the "miracle vitamin" because of its ability in the body to improve overall health. Vitamin D is believed to help prevent autoimmunity. Autoimmunity is when cells of your immune system fight healthy cells of the body. Although it's not the only measure to prevent for autoimmunity however, the immune system does suffer in the absence in Vitamin D.

Vitamin D accomplishes this by not triggering or arming T cells. T cells can attack the tissues of the body when they are activated by proteins, which means that the T-cell will recognize the native protein as being foreign. This kind of attack could ultimately lead to the growth of cancers that may be fatal. This is why Vitamin D is said to assist in the prevention of cancer.

Because Vitamin D is essential for the health of our immune system, it helps in reducing the incidence of a variety of ailments like influenza. By strengthening immunity, regardless of event of an outbreak the person is less prone to contracting the disease.

Vitamin D is thought to boost the effectiveness in your body's immune system by an number from 3-5. It also boosts the production of powerful anti-microbial proteins. They are exactly the proteins that your body requires in order to combat a huge variety of illnesses.

Vitamin D and Heart Disease

Researchers are now discovering that Vitamin D insufficiency can cause chronic heart failure (CHF), cardiovascular disease peripheral arterial disease, and heart attacks. The minimum daily intake of Vitamin D is believed to be an important factor in decreasing the risk of developing heart disease.

Vitamin D can reduce the risk to develop heart problems because it reduces the risk of metabolic illnesses like hypertension and diabetes. It also helps in lessening inflammation, reducing the thickening of arterial walls, and decreasing the chance of hardening or calcification in the arterial walls.

136

Anyone who starts to consume the recommended amount of Vitamin D as they are young will dramatically reduce the risk of developing cardiovascular disease when they grow older.

Vitamin D and Pregnancy

The most emotional moment in a woman's life can be when they are expecting and is preparing to welcome another human being to the world. It is during this time that the majority of women take extra care of their nutrition needs since they know that there is a person who is completely dependent of them in terms of their growth and development.

To to build up the baby's teeth and bones, the body requires Vitamin D to assist in its absorption of calcium as well as the phosphorus. If there is a deficiency, the infant could be afflicted with problems throughout life and may experience an enlargement of the skeleton, or a slowing of growth. This can be observed with low birth weight and also in low birth weight.

If a child is lacking Vitamin D at birth, the child is at a higher chance for developing the rickets. In this early age, it could result in deformities due to fractures as bones aren't strong enough to withstand simple movement. In certain instances growth and physical maturation of the child could be delayed. The deficiency could have an effect that lasts for the rest of his life on the development of bones in children and immune system.

For moms who are expecting the natural birth could be not possible due to a deficiency in Vitamin D has been linked to preeclampsia, which can lead to an early, unplanned birth of the baby via an obstetrical caesarean.

It is suggested that pregnant women take in four thousand IU in Vitamin D every day on a regular basis, particularly if cannot spend their time outdoors in the direct sun. The amount of Vitamin D should rise slightly, maybe up to 6000 IU a day in the case of lactation.

Women are frequently prescribed prenatal supplements to cover the absence of any vitamin when they become pregnant. But, they usually don't contain a sufficient level of Vitamin D and, therefore, the addition of the consumption of a Vitamin D high-fat diet as well as getting exposure to the sun are highly suggested. However, it is important to note that a physician is always recommended prior to using any supplements.

Vitamin D and sleep

Parents often inform to their kids that they develop while they sleep. The body is constantly working in a variety of ways even while you're asleep. So, it's not a wonder to learn that Vitamin D is required by your body while you are asleep and relaxing.

A lot of people suffer from sleep disorders of different types, and they generally impact the quality of sleeping. Certain people are unable to sleep, others suffer from sleep apnea and others have trouble sleeping and etc. These problems are typically due to a lack of nutrients in the body.

The consumption of Vitamin D is linked to the body's capacity to ensure a good night's rest. The more intake of Vitamin D is, the less chances of suffering in sleeping soundly.

Chapter 21: Vitamin D And Mental Health

Vitamin D is a great option for treating a wide range of physical ailments and issues within the body, which includes those that affect the body's tissues and cells. Apart from these physical ailments, Vitamin D is also capable of helping with mental illnesses to boost well-being and can lead to feeling better.

In general, Vitamin D has been connected to assisting in the treatment of depression, as explained within this section.

Vitamin D and depression

The pressures of life's daily routine have resulted in an increase of depression across the globe. The term "depression" refers to a psychological illness which affects the mood of a person. In the present, depression is prevalent among people of all ages, regardless of social status or backgrounds. Individuals suffering from depression might feel depressed unhappy, angry, or frustrated for extended periods of time.

If not treated depression and its symptoms can seriously affect the day-to-day life, causing them to be unable to move the point that they're unable to take any choices, be focused on anything or even feel joy in any way.

Vitamin D is a key role in the treatment of mental health problems and their treatment. It was discovered it is believed that Vitamin D can act on the brain regions which are associated with depression, however more research needs to be conducted to discover the exact mechanism behind this.

There are a variety of angles connecting the lack in Vitamin D to an increase in depression-related symptoms. The first one is connected the sun exposure. There are some people who have depression issues because they don't spend enough time outside. But, scientists are trying to come to a consensus on a single issue: whether a deficiency of Vitamin D is the cause of depression, or depression results from a deficiency in Vitamin D.

Vitamin D is a key component in chemically fighting depression. This is connected to the fact that this Vitamin is great to the brain. Vitamin D helps regulate dopamine, noradrenaline, and adrenaline manufacturing in the brain. This is accomplished through Vitamin D receptors that can be located within the cortex of adrenaline. Additionally, Vitamin D offers protection against the depletion of serotonin and dopamine. A rise of 8 to 14 percent in depression has been linked with those suffering from an Vitamin D deficit.

Researchers have also attempted to determine if there is a link with Vitamin D deficit and suicidal behavior. It was found that low concentrations in Vitamin D could increase the likelihood of suicide. The next phase of research is to determine if the increase in Vitamin D levels may be beneficial to treatments for depression.

Vitamin D as well as Schizophrenia

As well as depression, the absence or deficiency in Vitamin D has also been connected to a mental disorder. Schizophrenia is a condition that can be seen in those with abnormal levels of Vitamin D in their systems. This is especially true for infants whose mothers did not consume sufficient amounts of Vitamin D while they were expecting. If the child is not diagnosed with schizophrenia, they're still susceptible to becoming afflicted as they age.

Chapter 22: Vitamin D And Weight

The people who are overweight or obese are believed to be at a higher risk of developing a Vitamin D insufficient. Although increased sun exposure and taking a daily supplement (recommended dosage) will help in reducing the problem but it's been discovered that their bodies aren't getting the amount that is needed. Therefore, it's crucial for someone who is obese or overweight to take a supplement in order to make up for a deficit. In these cases, the powerful Vitamin D3 supplements are recommended.

People who are overweight have difficulty release Vitamin D from their skin. It is believed that this happens due to the fact that the fat beneath the skin holds on to Vitamin D which is fat soluble.

Additionally, gender is an factor which affects Vitamin D as well as weight loss, particularly when it comes to weight gain or loss. Women typically are more fat-laden than men, andconsequently, they have a slower release of

Vitamin D through the skin, as well. In women, a portion part of Vitamin D will be transported to the liver to process, while others will stay in fat cells which is where the signal will be transmitted to them for them to store.

Supplements are taken on an everyday, weekly or even monthly basis. The amount to be consumed is dependent on the dosage that is recommended by a doctor. If someone's goal is to make sure they're getting all the nutrients that are present in your body, it is recommended to consume the most minimal amount they can get and take it in one dose each daily.

Anyone suffering from a deficiency must be sure to check your Vitamin D levels at least every 2 to 3 months after beginning treatment. In excess of the upper limit of recommended Vitamin D can cause damage to the kidneys and tissues. It may also result in significant increases in the levels of haemoglobin AIC as well as C-reactive protein. The worst-case scenario could be a rare instance that is a result of Vitamin D toxicity.

Vitamin D and weight loss

Research supports the idea of Vitamin D may be good news to lose weight. It was discovered that each kind of cell in our body requires Vitamin D. That is also applicable to fat cells, those that the majority of people seek to eliminate once they start their weight loss plan.

Vitamin D is well-known for its ability to attach itself to cell receptors and influencing the signals or messages that cells transmit. This Vitamin D signal is able to communicate whether the body needs to burn fat, or whether weight should remain stored. The receptors typically suggest that fat must be burned, and the faster they burn, the increase the chance of losing weight.

Furthermore there are also receptors in the brain that aid to reduce hunger cravings and cravings. They also aid in helping to improve moods as they may increase levels of serotonin, a chemical. Vitamin D can give them the appropriate signals, which help limit the urge to eat, and also to prevent depression which could cause emotional eating.

In terms of Vitamin D assisting with weight loss, it boosts the body's capacity to absorb nutrients crucial for weight loss for instance calcium. If a body has a shortage of calcium (in the case that it's not effectively taken in) is likely to have an increase of five times than the normal amount of Fatty Acid Synthase. This is a problem since it is the enzymes in this acid convert the calories to fat.

Injecting Vitamin D in the body could trigger the body to shift into a burning state instead of an accumulation of fat. This can accelerate the loss of weight by around 70 percent.

Chapter 23: Understanding Where Vitamin D Fits In The Paleo Diet

The Palo Diet has received an immense amount of attention and has garnered a massive and loyal following in recent times. This Paleo Diet is focused on being healthier through eating healthy foods, including healthy meats, vegetables fruit, nuts, and other vegetables. It's not strict regarding portions, and it doesn't need to keep the list of every item one consumes or keeping track of calories. It also eliminates food items that aren't in their original forms and were not consumed in time during the Paleolithic period. The theory behind this is that more than 10,000 years ago our diet did not include any processed or junk food items. The argument is that our bodies haven't yet adjusted to the diet changes that have taken place in the wake of Industrial Revolution, and we do not like food items that have been processed, or that contains sugars or grains.

The reason why the diet is so popular is that a lot of people have realized that they can alter their eating habits while still enjoying eating food and losing weight in the process.

One downside of Paleo Diet is that it lacks Vitamin D. Paleo Diet, though, is the absence amount Vitamin D.

There is an imbalance in vitamins and minerals in this diet, as certain nutrients are in high quantities while others aren't there at all, or are present in extremely small amounts. For instance it is possible to get an array of B vitamins as a result of eating leafy greens as well as meat and fish. There could be excessive amounts of sodium from animal protein sources. Calcium might be absent in this diet since the majority of people get their calcium through dairy products or cereals that are fortified. It is also difficult to find sufficient Vitamin D. Foods which contain artificially fortified Vitamin D are usually processed grains, cereals and milk, but they aren't consumed as part of this diet.

Paleolithic man had plenty of Vitamin D due to spending much time in the sun while gathering and hunting. Also, the human body produces Vitamin D when exposed to sunlight. It's a different story for people today. Our modern lifestyles are centered around spending the majority of time in buildings or vehicles, which means that individuals are likely to spend very little or even no time outside on a regular basis. The fact that they do not spend much hours in the sun and not eating food items that are rich in Vitamin D indicates that a person who follows The Paleo Diet is likely to be deficient in this Vitamin.

In any diet, it's important to be aware of all the nutritional components of the diet. In the event that you realize that this diet doesn't provide enough Vitamin D even with all the fresh produce and vegetables it is possible to make a decision to add a supplement for the body to perform optimally.

Chapter 24: Vitamin D And Lifestyle

Since Vitamin D is at the forefront and there are many discussions and research projects in progress to learn more about it, it's essential to fix the damage that has already been caused. This means focusing on reversing the problems caused by deficiency to allow people to live more healthy lives. The best method to accomplish this is to look at lifestyles and ways to be improved or changed.

Insufficient time spent outdoors in the Sunlight

Many people are suffering from Vitamin D deficiency because they don't spend enough time in the sunshine. It is easiest to understand this by looking at an example of what an average person does in one day.

If a person is starting with their workday, they might be on a journey to work, and they travel in a bus, train or in a car. They spend the rest of the day working in front of a laptop all day long until the sunset. Even if they're able to open their windows during work, they'll usually be closed to stop the wind from blowing away valuable documents.

When the day, a person is expected to leave work and travel to home, typically at sunset.

There isn't much time in the day to soak up the sunshine. On weekends, the person could be lying in the morning while finishing household chores during the remainder time. Also, there isn't much time spent outside in the sun.

It is possible that this person will come alive in the evening, attending the nightclub or out for dinner with friends to have an enjoyable time. In a flash the months could go without spending time in the sun.

If this person faces the additional challenge of living in an area in which there is a long winter that leads to a lower amount of sunshine than usual the chances are they're going to suffer from the Vitamin D insufficient.

This requires a shift of lifestyle completely. The most optimal time to enjoy sunshine to create Vitamin D creation is that in the middle of the day. Therefore, it is recommended to take your lunchtime in the sun, taking advantage of the sun as they take advantage of their midday meals.

Additionally, those living in areas that have only a little sunlight must be sure to take advantage as they can from the summer season. People with light skin tone can set a goal of spending just 10 minutes per day to boost the Vitamin D levels. On the other hand people with darker skin tone and older can set a goal of spending 30 minutes a day in the sunlight.

In the winter months, when sunlight is scarce all people should be encouraged to consume supplements regularly to satisfy the body's requirements of Vitamin D. This has to be considered routine instead of an supplement to a diet already in place.

Consuming a Diet that isn't balanced

What we put into our mouths for nourishment plays a crucial impact on your overall wellbeing. With the growing number of obese and overweight people around the globe It is evident that a large portion of the food we consume is not healthy.

Ingestion of unhealthy foods could lead to a wide range of ailments that impact the body.

When these conditions occur, there's more strain on the body's ability to absorb Vitamin D and, If a person isn't getting enough vitamins to manage the pressure, they can be afflicted with the Vitamin D deficit.

It's time to transform the way you live your life, which revolves around convenience foods and junk food, as well as fast food and fried food in a way that's sensible and healthy, in order to ensure a balanced supply of minerals, vitamins and nutrients within the body.

There are some diets that try to accomplish this, like those that advocate the Paleo Diet, but even these diets aren't enough in terms of Vitamin D. No matter what type of diet you decide to follow it is essential to be aware of all options for Vitamin D available in order to know whether you need to supplement your diet.

In order to ensure that your diet contains lots of Vitamin D it is essential to include eggs, milk as well as salmon, liver as well as fortified grains in ample quantities. Foods with calcium must also be eaten so that Vitamin D will work in conjunction in conjunction with the mineral, which can prevent it from sinking and growing inside a fat cells.

While an eating plan that is packed of Vitamin D-rich food does not assure that you'll be able for you to fulfill the minimal requirements daily, these foods could help bridge the gap due to insufficient Vitamin D doses through the sun or supplements.

A new way of living through spending more time in the outdoors as well as taking in more Vitamin D food items will make a huge difference in improving your overall health. A better understanding of your diet is essential to ensure that you've covered all the nutritional needs.

Chapter 25: Fantastic Tips On How Vitamin D Makes You Feel Great

The book attempts to provide all the information you should learn regarding Vitamin D. This final chapter will highlight the many benefits of Vitamin D, and how when you are getting the proper amount, you will be able to have more fun since you'll feel amazing.

Have Strong Bones - If you have the chance to meet someone experiencing bone problems like osteoporosis You will be able to feel a new appreciation of having healthy bones. With strong bones, you can comfortably engage in all kinds of sports and feel more balanced, without joint pain, and amazing posture. Vitamin D will help you feel this as a constant experience.

Aids in maintaining healthy Hair It is the result of the spillover effect from other benefits. Vitamin D intake has been linked to reducing stress levels. Additionally, this means there is less chance of losing hair. Healthy hair has been discovered to be a source of Vitamin D in the follicles. Hair that is unhealthy does not contain Vitamin D in its hair follicles.

Enhance your Teeth Your smile can be an amazing gift to give to others and it's even more attractive if you've got stunning teeth to display. As calcium is required for bones, it's necessary for teeth. in conjunction with Vitamin D solid teeth will be the norm of the day.

Directly to the brain. Vitamin D helps brain functionality and keeps you focused and alert as you age. It can aid you in all areas of your life, as well as the way you interact with other people. Imagine how rich your conversations will be if you keep track of the little things. Vitamin D is very helpful for this purpose.

Helps with all of the cells inside your body are created to function as a machine to maintain maximum efficiency. But, all machines require some oil from time to time to function properly. Vitamin D is the oil that helps your cells. In helping provide nourishment to your cells, you reap the benefits of preventing disease and better cell functionality. Plus, your mood could improve and you'll be able to be more peaceful and more positive.

Protect yourself for Certain Diseases - Have you noticed that there's an outbreak of influenza? If you have a high level of Vitamin D in your body, you are less likely to contract the highly contagious flu. It can be due to the fact that your body's equipped to fight illnesses and even autoimmune disorders.

It helps prevent cancer Vitamin D is recognized to prevent certain types of cancer. While this is a marginal benefit in its nature, the fact that it is available gives people the chance to create the best protection against cancer.

Chapter 26: What Is Vitamin D Is And Why You Should Have It

"Vitamin D is interesting because it isn't only a part of the "vitamin" category, but it is also a good fit in the "hormone" category as well. It's actually the precursor to a hormone called steroid that's created by UV-B radiation from the sun that strike the surface of your body." Source The Amazing Wonder Nutrient that could help prevent or treat seven common diseases - written By Dr. Mercola According to Dr. Mercola, one of the most renowned medical researchers As high as 88% of people are in danger of being deficient or low of vitamin D. Because vitamin D acts as both an essential vitamin and a hormone within the body, its absence is a cause for various diseases and illnesses. These numbers aren't getting better as more research is conducted. This isn't just a problem this country, nor across the United States, but worldwide. Studies have shown that a lot of ailments caused by vitamin D deficiencies can be prevented or even being cured (source Mercola above) if appropriate diet modifications and supplements are followed.

So what exactly is Vitamin D as a "Formula?" Vitamin D as we have mentioned previously is a fat-soluble vitamin that belongs to a family of vitamins. It is typically found in eggs, liver yolks, yeastand and even wool from sheep, and/or fish oils. Vitamin D is crucial for getting calcium into your body. it functions as a potent hormone in the body . It actually plays a role in the prevention of a variety of ailments, particularly osteomalacia in children, and rickets in adults. The body is brimming with vitamin D receptors, which aren't connected with the utilization of calcium or phosphorous. This is a proof of the way vitamin D can affect the entire body. What exactly is vitamin D? It's actually a mix of two elements: Vitamin D2 is commonly called calciferol. The vitamin D3 is usually called the cholecalciferol. Remember that vitamin D actually a blend of both cholecalciferol as well as calciferol. Similar to the B vitamins vitamin D, in its purest form is thought of as blended. The finest vitamin D blends function synergistically within your body, yet it is bio-active Lee in its art form until it undergoes changes within the body to make it work effectively. What happens to the body with Vitamin D? Vitamin D can be first processed in the liver , and then converts into what is known as vitamin hydroxy D or calcidiol. The second form of conversion is found in the kidney , where the substance begins to become active. It is known as the calcidiol. The vitamin is then distributed throughout the body. This is the time that the body can making use of it for the absorption of calcium and phosphorous. Bones are strengthened, and bone growth could occur. It is important to remember that this is just the beginning as this body released substance functions as an effective hormone. This permits both calcium and phosphates for calcium and phosphates to strengthen your bones and to also prevent bone-related diseases. You need to be able to get enough amounts of Vitamin D otherwise you may develop brittle and even sagging bones, particularly during the formative years as well as in older years. Vitamin D is a crucial ingredient in protecting seniors from osteoporosis, and to aid children and teenagers to grow in a healthy way. Pros and Cons of Vitamin D

Vitamin D is an essential function in the body. It is involved in many other activities that we'll discuss in this article. We will just declare that it is essential for every stage of development, and later in life to keep well-being and good health. Vitamin D, in particular the more potent forms of vitamin D, aren't typically found in the standard diet. It is more than adding dairy products to your diet in order to receive the best high-quality vitamin D. Although vitamin D is produced by the body through sunlight exposure on the skin it is the simplest form of vitamin D that can help you stay well, but it may not be enough to stop the reduction of bone mass or health problems. The skin exposure to absorb vitamin D is only one piece of the equation. To stay healthy and enhance overall wellness, it is essential to add vitamin D, to your diet and have the right levels of exercise and sun exposure for your skin. This is exactly what we're going to discuss in this article so that after you've finished reading, you'll be aware of everything you have to know to stay in good health, and that includes the right introduction of vitamin D from the sun into your diet and to your daily life. This guide will also discuss the the proper levels of concentration, as well as best supplements, and how to identify high quality vitamins and what are low quality vitamins. Due to the depletion of the amount of nutrients found in mass-produced food as well as junk food as well as other non-nutritious diet supplements, it's crucial to investigate these issues to alter and modify the amount of vitamin D you consume in the proper amounts. It is possible to consume excessive amounts of vitamin D, which could cause adverse negative effects, and could even cause health problems. Vitamin D is a vital role to play in the daily life. It is crucial to learn more about this vitamin as your capacity to keep your health, the proper function of joints, and the strength and health of your bones will determine the level of activity you can keep up as you age. Unsuitable quantities of vitamin D, or the improper types of vitamin D may contribute to health problems too. We'll go over this in a little more detail later in this article. It is of paramount importance that young and elderly are taking vitamin D supplements also. Both require additional requirements and ought to be given priority even the amounts of vitamin D among the young people were higher than those of adults. This is because the formative years are crucial to bone development as well as future wellbeing and health. In the end, deficiency rates depend on blood glucose readings that reveal persistent deficiency. The CDC is a devoted researcher and we will refer to these sources and indices when we investigate the appropriate levels of supplements to address deficiencies. Then we will look into what will happen to those who don't take precautions against deficiencies. We will also look at what may occur to them, even if they're aware of what it means.

Chapter 27: What Is A Nutrient?

There is a lot of talk regarding nutrition, and some even eat "nutrient rich" foods. What exactly is an nutrients? What is its significance for our bodies? What are the tasks it plays in our body?

Simply put, a nutrient considered to be a part in the food items that living creatures require to survive and grow.

Nutrients are broadly classified into twocategories:

Macronutrients These are the major weights that supply the body with the energy needed to perform the different metabolic functions. The body needs these nutrients in large amounts.

Micronutrients: Although not essential micronutrients, they supply the body with cofactors (i.e. the essential nutrients) that aid in the working of the metabolic processes. The need for these nutrients is not as high and they should be consumed in smaller amounts.

Both, macronutrients as well as micronutrients are easily found in the world. They serve a multitude of roles to play within the body. They supply the body with energy, aid in the regulation of the bodily functions and assist in the creation of new tissues as well as fixing damaged ones.

Animals and plants have various methods of absorbing elements from the surrounding. The plants absorb the necessary nutrients from the soil by their roots, while leaves absorb elements from the air.

Animals have digestive systems that break down the food consumed and extracts macronutrients as well as micronutrients. The macronutrients are used to boost energy levels, while micronutrients aid in the execution of different metabolic functions within the body.

Organic Nutrients: Proteins vitamins, carbohydrates and fats

Inorganic Nutrients: Water oxygen, and minerals in dietary supplements.

That's the basic definition of the term "nutrient. Every thing we eat is made up of at least one or more nutrients in it, with some being greater than the others. In order to keep our bodies healthy, it is essential to eat various nutrient-rich food items to ensure that the body is nourished with all the nutrients needed to perform metabolic functions.

If you consume junk food such as French fries, the only thing the body gets is sugars, carbs, and sodium. The body receives energy from food, but since junk food isn't rich in micronutrients your body is unable to complete metabolic processes and that energy is wasted.

Recently, experts discovered that if you meet the requirements of both macronutrients as well as micronutrients is not a guarantee that one will live a long and healthy life. This was proven by the growing number of various diseases that are prevalent in west. The proportion of those who suffer from heart ailments or cancer as well as weight gain is too high these countries.

The reason is the rising quantity of junk food consumed in people's diets as well as the decreasing amount of physical activities. A balanced, healthy diet must always be coupled with some form of exercise to keep you fit and healthy for the rest of your the rest of your life.

The most important nutrients

All nutrients are essential, however, certain nutrients are more crucial than others.

A majority of people are able to consume adequate amounts of nutrients just by chance however, they aren't aware of the exact proportion of nutrients required to grow.

Every day every person is either using or losing a certain quantity of nutrients when performing various activities. In the event of an absence of a certain nutrients in the body tissues in the body utilize the stored nutrients to meet the requirements. However, if the proper nutrients aren't stored and consumed in the body, it will result in an absence of nutrients which can lead to deficiency.

As we have mentioned, certain nutrients play a much more significant function in our bodies. Here are a few nutrients that play an significant role in the body:

(a) Proteins

The word comes from an Greek word that means that it is the first position. Proteins are the basis for the development of an organism. Proteins are made up of amino acids, and are considered to be the primary components of the human body.

Protein is mostly found in milk, butter bread, cereals, bread and even meat. Vegans consume proteins from legumes, fruits and vegetables, as well as other dairy products. Vegans typically get their protein from soy-based products.

(b) Fats

The most important characteristic in fat is they aren't liquid in water, however they dissolve in organic substances known as Acetone. The texture of fat is oily and it is non-volatile. Fats aid in the performance of bothmetabolic and structural functions in the body.

Health experts explain fats in two ways, i.e. visible and invisibly. These are the fats that can be seen which are visible to our naked eyes. They include butter, olive oil cheese, sunflower spread, as well as the fat contained that are found within meat chunks. Invisible fats are those like sweets, junk food, egg yolks and more. Where you physically can't see the fat content of the item.

(c) Carbohydrates

Carbohydrates are a set of compounds that are typically found in both animals and plants. Although they aren't an essential element of nutrition but they are thought to be vital since they are among the primary sources of energy for our bodies.

Carbohydrates can be found in many different foods such as cereals, vegetables and pulses, dairy products and more. The majority of carbohydrates are present in processed food items.

(d) Vitamins

Vitamins are thought to be organic substances that play an essential role in many bodily metabolic processes. Vitamins could be water soluble or fat liquid, depending on the amount of chemical build-up.

There are 14 vitamin known as well as some most abundant source of them include lean meats, dairy products and green leafy vegetables. orange and yellow fruits, as well as vegetables.

What is A Vitamin?

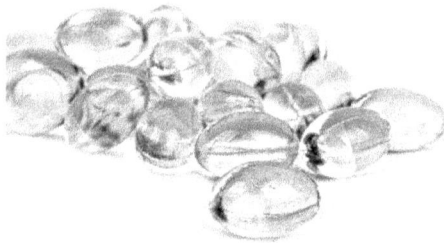

A vitamin is said as an organic compound that is necessary for development and growth and is needed in tiny amounts by our bodies. There are 13 vitamins that are recognized across the world in the present. They have a range of purposes to fulfill and the absence of these vitamins can cause deficiency-related diseases to the body.

Vitamin A also known as retinol , or retinal. Fat-soluble. In soy milk, orange and pumpkin. It is also found in carrots and yellow fruits, leafy veggies and many more.

Deficiency of night vision

Vitamin B1: Also referred to as Thiamine. Water soluble. It is found in liver, eggs, vegetables brown rice, pork oatmeal, potatoes, and many more.

Deficiency: Beriberi

Vitamin B2 Also known as Riboflavin. Water soluble. It is found in popcorn, green beans as well as asparagus dairy products, bananas and many more.

Deficiency: Ariboflaviosis

Vitamin B3: Also referred to as Niacin. Water soluble. It is found in fish, mushrooms trees, eggs, tree nuts meat, and other vegetables.

Deficiency: Pellagra

Vitamin B5: Also referred to by the name panthothenic acid. Water soluble. It is found in avocados, broccoli and even meat.

Deficiency: Parasthesia

Vitamin B6 is also referred to as pyridoxine, or pyridoxal. Water soluble. In bananas, in vegetables and tree nuts, as well as meat.

Deficiency: Anemia peripheral neuropathy.

Vitamin B7: Also referred to as biotin. Water soluble. It is found in peanuts, eggs, liver raw egg yolks, the green leaves of vegetables.

Deficiency: Dermatitis

Vitamin B9: Also referred to as Folic acid. It is found in liver, bread cereals, pasta, and many leafy veggies.

Deficiency: A deficiency in pregnancy causes birth defects

Vitamin B12 also called cyanacobalamine. It is present in meat as well as other products made from animals.

Deficiency:Megaloblastic anemia

Vitamin C is also called ascorbic acid. In high amounts in citrus fruits as well as many vegetables, and in the liver of animals.

Deficiency: Scurvy

Vitamin D also called the cholecalciferol (D3) or the ergocalciferol (D4). Fat-soluble. In mushrooms, eggs fish, and liver.

Deficiency that causes Rickets and Osteomalacia

Vitamin E also called tocopherols. Fat-soluble. In nuts, seeds fruits, and even vegetables.

Deficiency: Abortions in females and men, as well as sterility.

Vitamin K Also called phylloquinone, or menaquinones. Fat-soluble. In eggs, spinach and liver.

Deficiency: Bleeding diathesis

Vitamins are extremely important since they assist in the growth and development of cells in living creature. The fetus takes in nutrients of the mother and grows over the course of time. The fetus requires specific nutrients and vitamins to develop of skin, bones muscles, and various organs. In the event that the mother's diet is lacking in a specific vitamin, the baby may not develop normally or develop a condition that can have a long-lasting impact for the baby.

However, excessive consumption of these vitamins could cause harm to your body as well. This is why it's crucial to take just the "just the right" quantity of vitamin needed by your body. Don't consume excessively and not less.

Vitamin D

The first research based in Vitamin D started from the illness of rickets. Rickets is a bone-related disease that usually manifests in infants and the early years of the child's life. In 1919 Sir Edward Mellanby proved that the illness is due to the deficiency of nutrition and also demonstrated that the condition could be treated with the aid of sunlight.

In several years, various scientists, through the use of various studies and experiments investigated the advantages of UV rays to children suffering from rickets . The research discovered that the nutrients derived from sunlight had a significant effect on children suffering from rickets.

Vitamin D is considered as a category of secosteroids that are fat-soluble in the natural world. This secosteroids group assists the intestine to absorb calcium, magnesium, iron zinc and phosphate.

For humans as far as they are concerned as far as humans are concerned, according to the research, cholecalciferol (vitamin D3) and ergocalciferol (vitamin D2) are extremely essential for growth and development goals. The body is unable to make these substances internally, so it is imperative that we attempt to incorporate vitamin D into our diets as well as expose our bodies to sunlight to make vitamin D within our bodies.

Different types of Vitamin D

There are many kinds of vitamin D, based on its chemical structure. The two most popular varieties of vitamin D are ergocalciferol (vitamin D2) and the cholecalciferol (vitamin D3). Simply vitamin D without a subscript is either cholecalciferol or ergocalciferol. Or even both. Vitamin D3 as well as Vitamin D2 together are known as calciferol.

In 1931 Vitamin D2's chemical makeup D2 was determined along with the structural structure that vitamin D3 was established in 1935, after studying the effect of 7 dehydrocholestrol's effect on UV Rays.

The various forms of vitamin D chemically identified as secosteroids. Secosteroids are thought to be steroids with one broken steroid bond within their rings.

The vitamin is split into different kinds according to their chemical composition

1. Vitamin D1

2. Vitamin D2

3. Vitamin D3

4. Vitamin D4

5. Vitamin D5

Factors that Influence The Production Of Vitamin D3 in the Body

Many biological influences can influence the production and production of Vitamin D3 in the body. The most significant of these are ageing, fashion of clothing, exposure the sun, the excessive use of sunscreen lotions diverse types of pollutants, and the various seasons. In all the possible reasons that cause pigmentation, the level of ageing is the primary one.

(e) The Degree of Pigmentation in Skin

A lesser amount of solar radiation as well as skin pigmentation are two factors that impact how we produce Vitamin D3. This is because of melanin, which is able to fight the 7 dehydrocholesterol and blocks the absorption of ultraviolate radiations, which are vital for vitamin D3 production in the body.

(f) Ageing

As you get older the skin begins to thin. This process is initiated when you reach the age of 20. The level of the seven-dehydrocholesterol keeps on increasing with your growing age, but the production of vitamin D3 does not increase due to the thinning skin. Young adults can produce approximately three times the amount of vitamin D than his or her peers. As time goes by the skin's thickness keeps shrinking, which results in lower production of vitamin D.

(g) Use of Sunscreen

It is crucial to apply sunscreen lotion whenever you go outdoors in the sun because it shields your skin from being burned as well as from illnesses like skin cancer. The primary problem with sunscreens is that they block good radiation which aid in the creation of vitamin D3 in your body.

(h) Seasons

The season also affects how vitamin D is produced within your body. In cold regions, seven dehydrocholesterol levels are high for a brief period. Since summers are brief, the seven dehydrocholesterol levels are high for a few days. However, in such a short period, it can be difficult to make Vitamin D3 in large quantities.

This is why many people living in such nations prefer to spend their time on the beach and becoming bronzed.

Benefits of Vitamin D

Vitamin D is required for the human body's many different functions. One of the most significant tasks that require vitamin D is the growth of bone. Vitamin D aids calcium in its ability to be absorbed by the body of all living thing, and, as we know, calcium is vital for the development of bone within the body.

In addition it is beneficial in the development and growth of heart muscles and fat tissues as well as brain cells. Vitamin D regulates various cell growth and expansion throughout the body. This is why it is an important nutritional element for our body.
Additionally it aids in the regulation of metabolism and the immune system functions occurring in the body.

In the last few years, vitamin D has seen a surge in popularity. Vitamin D has led experts to engage in a constant debate. Certain studies suggest that vitamin D alone has no effect in particular, however when it is linked to other processes, it's highly beneficial.

www.ingramcontent.com/pod-product-compliance
Lightning Source LLC
Chambersburg PA
CBHW060332030426
42336CB00011B/1304